cannabis consulting

cannabis consulting

Helping Patients, Parents, and Practitioners
Understand Medical Marijuana

ezra parzybok

ForeEdge

ForeEdge
An imprint of University Press of New England
www.upne.com
© 2018 ForeEdge
All rights reserved
Manufactured in the United States of America
Designed by Mindy Basinger Hill
Typeset in Garamond Premier Pro

For permission to reproduce any of the material in this book,
contact Permissions, University Press of New England, One Court Street,
Suite 250, Lebanon NH 03766; or visit www.upne.com

Names: Parzybok, Ezra, author.

Title: Cannabis consulting: helping patients, parents,
and practitioners understand medical marijuana / Ezra Parzybok.

Description: Lebanon NH: ForeEdge, [2018] |
Includes bibliographical references and index. |

Identifiers: LCCN 2018002870 (print) | LCCN 2018004236 (ebook) |
ISBN 9781512602869 (epub, pdf, & mobi) | ISBN 9781512601107 (pbk.)

Subjects: LCSH: Marijuana—Health aspects. | Marijuana—Therapeutic use. |
Cannabis—Social aspects.

Classification: LCC RM666.C266 (ebook) | LCC RM666.C266 P39 2018 (print) |
DDC 615.3/23648—dc23

LC record available at https://lccn.loc.gov/2018002870

5   4   3   2   1

In addition to [the] problem of comparable potency and [chemical makeup], there is the problem of set and setting. Experienced laboratory investigations as well as users of marijuana know that the effects of this drug are influenced by the physiological characteristics and condition of the individual, by his psychological makeup and state, by his reasons for using the drug, by his fantasies about the effect of the experience, and by the physical and social factors that define the setting in which the drug is used or administered. The situation is even more complicated than this. It is a principle of psychopharmacology that the effect of any single substance may vary with the route of administration.

LESTER GRINSPOON | *Marijuana Reconsidered* (1971)

Contents

Acknowledgments

I would like to thank everyone who supported me throughout the process of writing this book—first and foremost, my wife Brooksley, who has clearly known me for many lifetimes. My children Sanza and Marzden, thank you for being brave. Sue and Bang, your unconditional support seems to know no boundaries. Ben and Jan, our Parzy talks and brainstorms were essential. Jordan Heller and Michael Teig, thank you for your friendship and intellect. To my readers: Jenni, for believing it was good and important even though you're my mom; Michelle, for your scientific perspective and encouragement; Rosie and Blair, for your deep and thoughtful feedback. I would like to thank my legal team of Richard Evans and Mike Cutler for your decades of work bringing justice to this cause and for negotiating my freedom. Thank you to David, Bruce, Alex, and Jason, as well as the doctors, practitioners, and colleagues who believed in my vision. I'd also like to thank the many citizens, clients, neighbors, journalists, and friends who took a risk to support me in my work. The letters and stories I have included in these pages are real (but with names disguised to protect people's privacy). The anecdotes and testimonials are essential in helping to bring a human element to the war on drugs, and I deeply appreciate the permission to include them. I have my art school education at the Rhode Island School of Design and Bard College to thank for teaching me how to learn the rules before I break them. Also thanks to my agent James Fitzgerald and to everyone at UPNE. And a special thanks to my editor Richard Pult, who was the ideal filter for making this book what it needed to be.

cannabis consulting

Introduction

Like tens of millions of Americans, many of whom also have children, mortgages, and day jobs, my wife and I would smoke a little weed on the weekends while we worked in the overgrown garden of our new home. I didn't discover the stress-relieving benefits of pot until my wife and I were married and in our thirties, but I always cringed to hear her stories of shady marijuana purchases from pot dealers. While we stood in our flower patch discussing the matter, she asked if I had any interest in trying to grow our own marijuana.

At the time, I was an art and science teacher at a small nonprofit school providing education and services to teen moms who had dropped out of high school. I was burned out from nearly a decade of low pay and disengaged students. With the birth of our first child and a monthly mortgage, the art career I had studied for in college and graduate school had faded to a daily grind. I would teach to skeptical students all day and come home to a demanding baby, an old house that needed work, and a basement art studio that was collecting dust. Although I held on to the romantic dream of becoming a successful artist, the idea of making an inanimate and often esoteric object and then putting it into a gallery or collector's home, where few people would ever see my work, was less inspiring by the day. I was a people person, and ultimately knew I wanted to have a more personal connection to my audience. I did love to teach and to help others, so I was also seeking a more tangible and humanitarian effect on my audience. The typical gallery experience may inspire viewers, but I worked with students and families who suffered every day. Art felt like a Band-Aid at best. My heart sought a cure.

I also didn't want to turn into a stoner, but for lack of inspiration in my art studio I did plant a cannabis seed in my basement. Within a few years, I discovered an art form that I believe can help humanity and still resides on the cutting edge of society's cultural evolution. The concept of growing cannabis, concocting remedies, and giving it to people who are fighting sickness, disease, pain, or malaise is both a radical idea and an ancient one.

Many people now come to me as the "expert" on medical marijuana, but it was neither a medical degree nor cannabis regulations in Massachusetts, where I reside, that shaped my expertise. I came to my competence by approaching the plant objectively, by caring about the people I serve, and by applying the traditional uses of the drug to my patients' ailments. Without forcing cannabis into a purely pharmaceutical model, I hope to reveal to the reader in states where it is still illegal that cannabis is far more benign than many prescription drugs, and that embracing it as a medicine will create a net benefit to the community. Any communities that do not embrace marijuana as a medical option are burdening their doctors and hospitals, increasing the suffering of patients, and putting undue stress on those who care for the infirm. And in states where it is now legal, I want to highlight the subtleties of medicinal cannabis that are often lost within the ill-informed medical debate and stereotypical pop culture that surrounds the drug. As states begin to legalize adult use, I believe the need for proper medical marijuana education is important if we want to carry on the tradition and necessity of using cannabis as medicine. To illuminate how I believe properly contextualized cannabis can fill the middle ground between herbal remedy and pharmaceutical pill, I will talk about its history and its interaction with our cells and consciousness within the context of my patients' unique stories, as I knowingly broke the law to help them.

Many doctors, citizens, and governmental representatives are aware that cannabis has merit, that the thousands of studies on its medical efficacy point to the need for loosening the draconian laws that punish otherwise law-abiding people for using it in the privacy of their homes. Physicians such as David Cassarett, a professor at Duke University School of Medicine and author of *Stoned: A Physician's Case for Medical Marijuana*, have witnessed the positive effects of the plant. When I read his book, I naively assumed that his stature in the medical community would sway the federal government to legalize it for medicinal purposes. But the federal government still maintains that it is a Schedule I dangerous drug with no medicinal value. *The Pot Book*, edited by Dr. Julie Holland, is a comprehensive look at all the data on cannabis, from medical efficacy to addiction. The evidence of its medicinal efficacy is so overwhelming in her treatise that surely the debate is settled.

But in working with my patients, I learned that medical data presented by cannabis-friendly doctors will not convince everyone of the merits of cannabis. As a practitioner of cannabis, I guide patients toward sustainable health, using properly formulated cannabis, with the goal of reducing their consumption of harmful medications, but I also advise chronic users who fear they are dulling their brains with it and need a break. Cannabis users, parents, patients, and those who care for them need experts they can trust who have experience with all the facets of cannabis that contribute to or hinder medical efficacy. A doctor recommending cannabis is just the first step in discovering the relief it can bring. Even if patients are lucky enough to live in a state where cannabis is legal—and they have found themselves returning home from a dispensary with a selection of cannabis products—the medicinal results of ingesting those products are not predictable. Relief from ailments, or even a pleasant evening, are not guaranteed.

My heart aches for the sick people who come to me having been chewed up and spit out of the conventional medical model. Some have tried cannabis but are unsure how best to use it. With no medical training, no big marijuana dispensary backing me, and a commitment to and compassion for my patients, I bring to them the radical idea that health and balance can be arrived at differently from the often-corporatized cannabis and pharmaceutical model they are accustomed to. Within the context of its illicit and medicinal history, as well as my empathic approach to patients, I want to recontextualize cannabis use free of societal constructs on both sides of the debate. I believe this will foster healing as well as reassure citizens who are wary of its legalization. Despite strict regulations in legal marijuana states, once a bag of cannabis product arrives at home, no regulation that purports to track the product from "seed to sale" (in an effort to protect communities from its "diversion" by employees of the dispensary) will ever ensure that the marijuana is ingested appropriately, let alone by the right person. When we adapt an informed approach to cannabis that takes into account the physical, emotional, and psychological health of patients, recreational users, and their families, its proper use will be far more likely.

The process by which I gained experience in treating people medicinally with cannabis was essentially a closed loop. Before my home-based "grow operation" was raided by police—National Guard helicopters with Drug Enforcement Administration (DEA) agents spotted plants growing on a second-floor deck in back of my home—I grew the plant myself, observed its physical attributes, and how those attributes contributed to different effects. Then, I created custom remedies for patients. Unlike most growers, I now believe one should grow plants not for how high they get you or how much weight they produce at harvest. My strains were selected for the specific ways in which they brought quality of life and symptom reduction to the user. I also collect data on its effectiveness from other patients I've come to know intimately and have treated as well. When I have all this information, I can better explain how an individual should use the remedy based on my knowledge about the patient's ailments and attitude.

I also seek helpful ways to frame my patients' expectation of the formulation as its effects are felt in the body. Without proper explanation by someone a patient trusts, one can merely feel *stoned* using cannabis (or feel nothing) and later dismiss it as useless. But sick people can alter their relationship with their ailments for the better when they understand the science and power of the plant as it relates to their specific conditions and lifestyle. When they reset their cultural perception of pot to neutral, I find that patients are more easily opened up to its bona fide healing properties. Preconceived notions can block a positive response to the drug.

I still want to analyze the clinical data that back up using cannabis for pain or other ailments. I have no intention of being a snake-oil salesman. But as with taking pharmaceuticals approved by the Food and Drug Administration (FDA), not every patient will have reduced pain from a medication proven scientifically to be effective for pain. For example, a study on long-term opiate use actually showed an *increase* of pain in some patients.[1] If the cannabis—and my explanation of how it should help—doesn't work, then so be it. But at least cannabis is not killing the patient with a fatal overdose or causing life-threatening side effects.

I have also seen patients who are on so many pills that they don't know where one pill's effect ends and another's side effect begins. I know the doctors are not intentionally hurting their patients by overprescribing, but the morale of the patient can deflate with each new pill prescribed. Some doctors (or cannabis dispensaries) have thousands of patients on their roster and see one for just a few minutes before filling out a prescription—or filling a baggy with pot. Many dispensaries or individual retail clerks do their best to foster a more intimate connection with patients, but often a lack of understanding of how the cannabis will affect the individual patient, strict regulations, or the sheer size of the dispensary can prevent the care a patient needs.

The pharmaceutical industry or large medical offices may require substantial infrastructure or administration to fulfill regulatory obligations or satisfy shareholders, but medical cannabis does not. For generations, home cannabis growers have safely grown, formulated, and provided remedies for their communities. Because the medicine is home grown does not necessarily mean that it is illicit or dangerous. Some succumb to cannabis harms, but it is an herb that cannot kill. The most immediate danger of cannabis is that of a user not understanding how to use it properly. Thus, some feel safer knowing the person who grows—and guides—their cannabis use. The grower can explain to them how potent it is or what ailment it is good for. They can begin a deeper conversation around healing that few patients get when interacting with doctors or pharmacists.

But imagine the synergy that occurs when a patient discovers how to literally grow the plant and formulate her own cannabis medicine at home. If she makes a remedy and sells it to a neighbor who also suffers, she's considered a drug dealer. Over more than a century, Americans creating their own therapeutic loop with cannabis have been considered criminals. Today in my state of Massachusetts, where we have legalized marijuana for adult use, she can still be charged with distribution of a controlled substance and sent to jail. The law requires it to be purchased from the heavily regulated dispensaries, where patients can wait in line for hours to acquire medicine from a retail clerk with no medical knowledge. Yet as I have heard many times from home growers and patients in similar situations, often the sickly neighbor still prefers to get cannabis privately from the person she trusts. This may not be the appropriate choice for everyone, but it should be allowed.

In yogic philosophy, there is the concept of the *rishi,* or Yoga devotee who has escaped from society to dedicate his life to Yoga. And then there is the Yoga householder. He or she uses Yoga to maintain health and balance while keeping a home, a career, and a family. I am not a dyed-in-the-wool devotee of cannabis. I am a cannabis householder, and parent, who wants to visit the pharmacy (as well as the cannabis cupboard) as little as possible. I am like the thousands of cannabis householders across the nation and world, but because I decided to make cannabis my public profession, and I proved to a prosecutor that my efforts were not harming my community, I can share our story.

If regulations allow dispensaries to serve informed users as well as individual home growers to sell cannabis from their small-scale farms, this will provide a wider spectrum of services for patients. My entire operation before I was busted by the DEA took up less than five hundred square feet in my home, yet it had served roughly two hundred patients. Many, like me, grow their prized medicinal strains secretly in their attics or basements, their medicinal remedies going to far fewer clients than I had as a professional cannabis consultant. The extra money they earn by selling the cannabis stays in the community and provides needed cash in a struggling economy. When dispensaries open in their towns, churning out marijuana to the thousands who line up to purchase it, the home growers who sell cannabis must still remain secret. The dispensaries may be replacing petty drug dealers, but armed guards and surveillance cameras that keep the cannabis safely locked in vaults are not necessarily addressing the harms of cannabis such as addiction and misuse when it leaves the building. Instead, the complex regulations governing dispensaries inadvertently criminalize caring citizens who love to garden, can privately help those in need, and may be better able to address the misuse and addiction of the people they serve. Because cannabis grows easily almost everywhere, what is needed is education and guidance for consumers, not more security guards and tracking systems.

Since I planted my first seed, I have always sought to help the people in my community by educating adults and their children about the actual harms and benefits of marijuana. Because I truly believe cannabis will provide a net benefit to communities, I still offer consultation to patients and practitioners on how to safely use it and other products such as cannabidiol (CBD), a legal constituent of cannabis. My story will show how I convinced the court that what I was doing not only was safe but was fulfilling a humanitarian need not entirely met by the current regulatory framework around cannabis. I will also answer the pressing questions about children and cannabis, but first I will explain how its complicated history informs the current debate. Regardless of its potential harms to children, its proper medicinal use by the adults who care for them will reduce the stress on the medical system and keep opioid addiction down. But first we must separate historical perceptions from current reality.

On the front lines of medical marijuana, people are relinquishing dangerous pills in favor of this medicinal plant. Many people ask me, What is the difference between medical and recreational marijuana? The short answer is context. It is the consciousness you, your provider, and your community bring to it when all the facts are considered. The same knowledge and service I have brought to my work can and should be offered at dispensaries, or it should be allowed to exist legally within the zoning regulations already in place for homeowners who sell produce they've grown at home. Regardless of how regulations ebb and flow over the years, if we want to empower our loved ones to embrace and understand the medicines that make them well, then we have a satisfying model in medical cannabis; we can grow it ourselves, prepare our own remedies, and advise others on how to find relief better than a bud tender behind a dispensary counter who has never met the patient before. When communities understand and witness the benignity of cannabis, perhaps then the military helicopters will stop flying overhead, looking for a particular medicinal plant to rip out of citizens' yards.

one

Confessions of a Cannabis Consultant

Visually speaking, the pot leaf is an iconic symbol, recognizable the world over. People who choose to adorn their clothing, their dorm rooms, or bodies with the pot leaf are presumably expressing passion for the subject, but as with the ubiquitous peace signs and popular religious symbols, it is difficult to separate the often shallow cultural construct of marijuana from the subtle, biological, and historical reality of the plant.

In the United States it is portrayed in music, TV, movies, and at the school nurse's office in roughly the same way: as a smokable plant that makes you space out. Very little is dedicated to the distinction between hemp, marijuana, and medicinal cannabis, let alone how its medicinal attributes can help one patient and hinder another. Displaying cannabis leaves on clothing and in imagery may be a way for users to come out of the closet. But it is literally a two-dimensional representation of a multifaceted herb that has been intertwined with human culture for thousands of years. To understand what is now the fastest-growing industry in America and pot's abilities to help or harm a user, it is important to get a sense of its ancient medicinal context, as well as the winding and often circular path it has taken from hemp to medicine to illicit drug in America.[1]

How Did We Get Here?

Cannabis is one of the oldest domesticated plants and can be traced back thousands of years, as it evolved agriculturally and medicinally alongside human culture. Although the biological origins of the plant are in Mongolia, the earliest written evidence of cannabis uncovered to date is from China roughly 4,500 years ago. Cannabis was grown for centuries in China for making paper, rope, and as a food source. It was also prescribed for ailments such as rheumatism, menstrual issues, and purportedly as an anesthetic in surgeries.[2] In 2006 cannabis was found in a basket and clay container in a 2,500-year-old tomb in Xinjiang, China. Because the tomb was a shaman's, it is speculated that the cannabis was used for ritualistic as well as medicinal purposes.[3] This points to its consciousness-shifting attributes, which blur the lines between physiological healing and emotional and psychological well-being. Anyone who has developed an ailment that the doctor says may be "stress related" is familiar with this concept. Unfortunately for China today, due to the fact that cannabis consumption and distribution is a crime punishable by imprisonment and possibly death, its medicinal connections in the country have been all but lost.

But in India, where law enforcement around the plant is less stringent, cannabis has an ancient and complicated medicinal history as well as modern uses. Its medicinal origins come from Ayurveda, the traditional medicine that has been passed down from teacher to student for over five thousand years. Ayurveda translates as "life knowledge" and utilizes more than two thousand medical formulations, mostly plant derived, in treating disease. Cannabis is referenced in Ayurvedic medical texts as far back as 1500 BCE.[4] But as some of the earliest medicinal origins of the cannabis plant point to northern India, some ethnopharmacologists speculate that human use of the plant in that region could go back tens of thousands of years.[5]

In Sanskrit, the original language of Ayurveda, the whole plant is referred to as *vijay*. *Ganja* refers to the resinous flowers, and *bhang* describes the leaves, which are easily collected from *vijay* growing in the wild. *Bhang* is also the name of a drink made with the leaves or any activated part of the plant that is traditionally consumed during the festival honoring the god

Shiva, reminding us that recreational and religious uses still intermingle for many who consume the plant. *Bhang* shops and Shiva worship flourish in modern-day India. Because the female plants provide the active resin, male and female cannabis plants were also separated by ancient Indian cultivators (as they were in China), and there are at least forty-three different synonyms for cannabis in Sanskrit texts.[6]

The varying synonyms from Sanskrit help explain the ancient as well as modern affinity for the plant. They also reflect the mixed results and debate surrounding cannabis that are observed in users today. For example, the cannabis synonym *tandrakrit* is defined as "causer of drowsiness" and obviously points to its now scientifically established sedative effects.[7] For a user unable to drag himself out of bed, this attribute could be a downside. For a patient with insomnia, it could be a lifesaver. Another Ayurvedic word describing cannabis, *capala,* translates as, "agile, capricious, mischievous, scatterbrained" and reflects the more recreational exploration of cannabis pursued by youth today. For a working adult, scatterbrained may be undesirable. For a person wanting to escape the stresses of working life, scattering one's thoughts and worries after a long day may be desirable. *Manonmana*—"accomplishes the objects of the mind"—might help an attention deficit/hyperactivity disorder (ADHD) sufferer unable to focus. I have met many medical marijuana patients diagnosed with ADD or ADHD who attest that cannabis is the only medicine that truly allows them to focus on the task at hand.

Ununda, "the laughter mover," obviously refers to the giggles many users experience while under the influence of the drug. Giggling in a college class may be untoward. Giggling with a loved one after a long battle with a terminal disease is a human right. I personally like *vrijapata,* "strong-nerved," as it points to the actions of cannabidiol (CBD), the second most prominent cannabinoid in cannabis. CBD is less psychoactive and a proven anxiolytic,[8] or antianxiety agent. I, along with many of my clients, take a nonpsychoactive form of CBD every day to keep anxiety at bay, cortisol levels lower, and to keep myself "strong-nerved."

Other words for cannabis in ancient India, such as *gatra-bhanga* or "body disintegrator," or *pasupasavinaini,* "liberates creatures from earthly bonds," may not be desirable results. Maureen Dowd, the *New York Times* columnist who wrote of her experience in Colorado eating a legally procured, cannabis-infused chocolate bar, articulated the feeling well: "I strained to remember where I was or even what I was wearing. As my paranoia deepened, I became convinced that I had died and no one was telling me."[9]

These Ayurvedic descriptions of cannabis are not scientific, as they were developed thousands of years before the scientific method became a standard practice in medicine. But they are not false. Over the millennia, patients and practitioners have experienced aspects of cannabis that are as diverse as the medicinal and recreational experiences of today. The language used to describe the varied aspects of the plant's effect on humans repeatedly points to our more emotional and psychological relationship with the plant. In short, response is unique to the individual. Thus, when clients come to me for guidance, I take into account their emotional and psychological state because it helps guide my choices in advising them how to safely pursue the myriad forms of medical marijuana.

Because effective medicinal herbs will be exchanged and shared by humans, it is not surprising that practitioners shared uses for cannabis throughout Asia, the Middle East, and Ancient Greece.[10] Assyrian clay tablets from the sixth century BCE have references to cannabis in the use of healing balms.[11] Cannabis was also known to be used in healing ointments in ancient Egypt.[12]

Some particularly poetic evidence has been found connecting the anointing practices in the Bible with cannabis. Although many translations for the word "cannabis" evolved throughout Middle Eastern languages and cultures, there is a pattern of treatment that emerges. In scripture, cannabis is often translated as aromatic, sweet or fragrant reed, cane, or stalk. And the word "Christ" is a Greek translation of the Hebrew word for Messiah, which means "anointed one." Anointing is to ritualistically apply oil to the body.

In Exodus 30:22, God gives an anointing oil recipe to Moses: "Then the Lord said to Moses, 'Take the following spices . . . liquid myrrh . . . fragrant cinnamon . . . fragrant cane [cannabis] and cassia. . . . Make these into a sacred anointing oil.'" In Mark 6:13, Jesus tells his followers to anoint the sick with oil: "They cast many devils, and anointed with oil many that were sick, and healed them." In James 5:13, James says, "Is any one of you sick? He should call the elders of the church to pray over him and anoint him with oil in the name of the Lord."[13] The researcher Chris Bennett synthesizes the biblical references to anointing oil for the purported miracles Jesus performed.

> Interestingly, cannabis has been shown to be effective in the treatment of not only epilepsy, but many of the other ailments that Jesus and the disciples healed people of, such as skin diseases (Matt. 8:1–4, 10:8, 11:5; Mark 1:40–45, Luke 5:12–14, 7:22, 17:11–19), eye problems (John 9:6–15), and menstrual problems (Luke 8:43–48). . . . Although the idea that Jesus and his disciples used a healing cannabis ointment may seem far-fetched at first, when weighted against the popular alternative (one that is held by millions of believers) that Jesus performed his healing miracles magically . . . the case for ancient accounts of medicinal cannabis seems a far more likely explanation.[14]

But as was discovered in India, not all responses to cannabis in Biblical times were positive. "To what purpose cometh there to me incense from Sheba, and the sweet cane [cannabis] from a far country? Your burnt offerings [are] not acceptable, nor your sacrifices sweet unto me" (Jeremiah 6:20).[15] It sounds as though Jeremiah may have had a bad trip similar to Maureen Dowd. Whether we're talking about an individual cannabis experience a thousand years ago, today, or a thousand years from now, I believe the issue will persist. Regardless of how successful we become at controlling its production or its action in the body, cannabis is difficult to dose and its effect is difficult to predict.

This inconsistency persists most strikingly in its history in America, which helps clarify why it occurs and why the legal pendulum regulating cannabis has swung to both extremes. Owing to hemp's practical uses for textiles, paper, and rope, in 1619 Britain decreed the growth of one hundred plants by individuals living in the American colonies.[16] Although there is essentially one species of *Cannabis sativa* (its proper botanical name), three different types of the plant have their own industries or cultures attached to them. *Cannabis sativa,* much the way *Canis familiaris* (the domestic dog), can be bred to create a myriad of different forms. Hemp is one. It usually contains very little in the way of medicinal resin but is bred to be a fast-growing, fiber-producing plant. The second form, marijuana, is essentially identical to *medical* marijuana yet is used in a different context. "Marijuana," a slang term originating from northern Mexicans who smoked it casually in the nineteenth century,[17] is currently bred to produce as much mind-altering resin per flower as possible. (If not for the war on drugs incentivizing growers to breed more potent plants in more confined spaces over the generations, marijuana would probably still be the mild stimulant it was in the 1960s.) The third form, medical marijuana, medical cannabis, or just cannabis, uses this same mind-altering resin but in a medicinal context. The cannabis-infused oil Jesus used is a good example of a medicinal use of the drug that does not produce a strong "high" because it is not ingested orally. There is another species (or subspecies, as it is still up for debate) called *Cannabis ruderalis,* which is common to very northern regions, but generally not a part of the medicinal conversation. I will exclude it from my comparisons. All versions of cannabis can cross-breed, but like canines, they have genetic differences.

At our country's inception, we find that the journals of both Thomas Jefferson[18] and George Washington reference their own hemp crops, and although Washington did separate the male and female plants,[19] pointing almost surely to internal consumption of some sort, there is no evidence that either smoked it. But within a single species planted in the garden, we begin to see how one person might be using it to make rope, aid his aches and pains, and take the edge off after a long day writing the United States Constitution.

It was not until 1839 that an exhaustive work on the medicinal attributes of cannabis was written by British doctor Sir William B. O'Shaughnessy, who translated the Ayurvedic, Persian, and Arabic medical texts he read as a physician in India.[20] Although hashish—a concentrated form of the resin—was readily smoked recreationally by the avant-garde in Europe,[21] O'Shawnessey is considered the first physician to apply the scientific method to his findings. His work inadvertently led to the bifurcation of medical and recreational cannabis into two parallel forms of consumption. As a result, medicinal cannabis was embraced by the European medical field and included in the *United States Pharmacopeia* from 1850 to 1940. He performed his own clinical trials, first on dogs, then on humans, and came up with his own parameters for proper dosing and titration using cannabis oils and tinctures.[22] O'Shaughnesy wrote of rabies sufferers whom he treated with the herb: "The influence of [cannabis], capable either of cheering or of inducing harmless insensibility, would be fraught with blessing to the wretched patient."[23]

We might assume that a doctor's scientific tests would properly clear up any confusion surrounding how to utilize it. But in the United States, this is where its use becomes increasingly complicated. With three very divergent applications of the plant, all coming from the same species, and no standard for production nor consistent separation of hemp from cannabis from hash from "loco weed," confusion prevailed. Pharmacies who sold it and physicians who prescribed it generally understood its myriad uses as medicinal *cannabis,* yet the medicine producers acquired it as *hemp* from India.[24] *Hash* was consumed recreationally by residents in cosmopolitan areas, but without any medical context for the hash consumption—and the fact that they were often grouped together with opium dens—hash dens were outlawed decades before the federal government removed cannabis from the *Pharmacopeia.*[25] Opium was also a prescription medicine at the time, but the banning of hash and opium dens was due in part to nationalist backlash against Chinese immigrants who often ran the opium dens, or Persian immigrants who ran the hash dens.[26] The first such statute was signed in Missouri in 1889 and stated that "every person who shall maintain any house, room or place for the purpose of smoking opium, hasheesh or any other deadly drug, shall be guilty of a misdemeanor."[27]

Although to this day there has been no reported fatality caused by the consumption of hash or any other form of cannabis, in 1866 a medical journal wrote warily of prescription hash candies (like marijuana edibles today) that were used "much more generally than is commonly supposed."[28] Frederick Hollick, a popular medical lecturer from Philadelphia, who grew and experimented with cannabis, also recommended it as an aphrodisiac in his *Marriage Guide* (New York, 1850).[29] It seems prescriptions for cannabis were as wide ranging and contextual then as they are today. It is not hard to conclude that an aphrodisiac for a married couple seeking guidance from a therapist has much different connotations than does one consumed by a sailor on leave who has just exited a hash den.

It is often believed that the 1937 Marihuana Tax Act was the beginning of the war on cannabis. But because of the culturally disparate uses, consuming cannabis without a prescription was made illegal in several states by the 1890s.[30] Unfortunately, with cultivation in North America now entering its fourth century, many varieties of wild-growing hemp were certain to contain more resin than others. Uninformed citizens could not tell the difference and began to be unnerved by foreigners or cosmopolitan youth using it in a nonmedical context. An 1897 article in the *San Francisco Call* reads, "In Southern Arizona the jail and prison officials have their hands full in trying to prevent the smuggling into their institution of the seductive mariguana [*sic*]. This is a kind of loco weed more powerful than opium. It is a dangerous thing for the uninitiated to handle, but those who know its users say it produces more raising dreams than opium. The Mexicans mix it with tobacco and smoke it with cigarettes, inhaling the smoke."[31]

Despite the government's creation of the 1906 Pure Food and Drug Act, which mandated the proper labeling of prescription drugs such as opium, cannabis, and cocaine by 1912, the confidence of pharmacists and chemists to properly prescribe cannabis was waning. A chemist wrote of his doubts in a trade publication, "Cannabis has fallen greatly into disuse in this country, and it matters little to us whether the drug is produced in Asia, Africa, or America. Quite possibly this lack of interest has been brought about by our failure to ensure that our preparations are always active."[32]

Paradoxically, the U.S. Department of Agriculture announced a year later that its pharmaceutical farms could successfully grow medical cannabis without foreign help.[33] Apparently, they didn't know that Middle Eastern immigrants to the United States had been successfully growing it to produce potent hash for decades.[34] Today this discrepancy persists in the fact that marijuana grown by the federal government for medical research purposes can come from only a single source: the University of Mississippi. The product it produces is known to be of a much lower quality than what is consumed in legal or illegal markets in the United States, making accurate research difficult.[35]

By the time the Marihuana Tax Act of 1937 was passed, requiring federal tax stamps for the possession of cannabis (further discouraging physicians and pharmacies from prescribing it), the public confusion surrounding the plant was well established. Jazz music was becoming popular in America and the counterculture that attended hash dens was now attending smoky jazz clubs, commingling with the diverse and rebellious youth from many backgrounds. Thus, the association with cannabis, foreigners, people of color, and illicit use was pervasive. When the beatnik and hippie cultures of the late 1950s and 1960s came along, the establishment attempted to squash the drug and its associated cultural forms. Even a 1944 report commissioned by the New York Academy of Medicine (known as the LaGuardia Report) that conclusively debunked many of the myths (that still persist today) about cannabis association with crime, as a gateway drug, or its addictive properties was condemned and deemed "unscientific" by Harry Anslinger,[36] the first U.S. commissioner of narcotics and architect of the Marihuana Tax Act.[37]

With the hippie era in full swing, President Richard Nixon had found another possible use for cannabis: winning elections. Although his family denies he said it, Nixon's domestic policy chief summed up the administration's antimarijuana efforts in a revealing 2016 *Harper's Magazine* interview: "We knew we couldn't make it illegal to be either against the [Vietnam] war or black, but by getting the public to associate the hippies with marijuana and blacks with heroin, and then criminalizing both heavily, we could disrupt those communities. We could arrest their leaders, raid their homes, break up their meetings, and vilify them night after night on the evening news. Did we know we were lying about the drugs? Of course we did."[38]

But as the hippie generation grew up, their brains intact for the most part, they could not deny the positive effects of cannabis. They still smoked it recreationally, but when a friend was nauseous or in pain, a relative was suffering from cancer treatment, or couldn't sleep, they knew what might help. Citizens risked breaking the law to bring relief because they observed its positive results and knew the side effects were less severe than those of many prescription medications.

In the 1970s, many states sought to reduce the penalties for cannabis or decriminalized the possession of small amounts. And finally, in 1996, in a great leap forward for sensible cannabis reform, a group of citizens, health practitioners, and state representatives in California successfully brought the state back in line with its 1913 cannabis laws.[39] They passed Proposition 215, which legalized the medicinal use of cannabis. Since the parallel cultures of medicinal cannabis and recreational marijuana hadn't been fully clarified (and probably never will be), the law enabled a mixture of both. As far as hemp is concerned, since the law was about human consumption of medical marijuana, this most benign form of *Cannabis sativa* was not addressed, even though the species is considered a superfood containing all nine amino acids and a protein content equal to or exceeding many nuts and grains.[40]

California state residents were allowed to acquire a doctor recommendation for the use of medical marijuana for "any illness for which marijuana provides relief . . . [that] if not alleviated, may cause serious harm to the patient's safety or physical or mental health."[41] From stress to insomnia, anxiety to depression, PMS to headaches, the definition was broad. Doctors were allowed to determine a patient's need but were not required to have any knowledge of cannabis, its proper use, dosing, or correct ingestion method. Because cultivation cooperatives were also legalized, you could create a one-stop marijuana dispensary if you could get a doctor to sit in a room and write recommendations to any resident who came in. As is the case in California and every other state with legalized marijuana today, retail clerks, growers, and business owners are not required to have any standardized knowledge of cannabis use for medicinal purposes.

This glaring lack of standardization or concern for patients contributed to many believing that medical marijuana legalization was just a Trojan horse for full legalization. For many proponents of the law who already knew how to use marijuana and were not especially sick, the law *was* a Trojan horse, and that was the point. They believed that whatever they did in the privacy of their home, medically or not, was their business. It's not to say the laws are lax. Regulations often require heavy security, databases of sales and products, software that tracks each gram of cannabis from seed to sale, strict lab testing, and childproof packaging requirements. But some regulations that do distinguish a clear difference between medical marijuana and recreational marijuana have backfired, in my opinion. For example, in Oregon, where cannabis is legal for recreational and medical purposes, the maximum percentage of the active ingredient tetrahydrocannabinol (THC) that products can contain is different for the two categories. Cannabis tinctures for recreational use can contain a maximum of 1,000 mg of THC, but for medical patients the maximum concentration is 4,000 mg.[42] If you're an average patient new to marijuana, 4,000 mg is far more than necessary to test a product for efficacy. A tincture of that concentration may last months, and the powerful effect from a single dose could scare a new patient away from medical marijuana indefinitely. Alternatively, if you're a recreational user with a high tolerance to THC who is comfortable being stoned all day long, the 1,000 mg tincture you're allowed to purchase may be a disappointingly small amount. There is no medical or scientific basis for this regulation, only perceptual.

Regardless of the discrepancies in potency, a typical dispensary providing medical cannabis will seek to answer questions posed by patients, as they may carry specific strains of cannabis or specific products that other dispensaries do not. This can also make standardization challenging. Thus, for some dispensaries, the 1960s traditions of community and sharing can create a culture that is more socially welcoming and educational than your typical hospital or doctor's office. Pot shops can be spaces where people chat and share stories and trade information about ailments. Bud tenders (the retail clerks in a dispensary) are often patients themselves and want to help others discover the benefits of the plant. Some dispensaries train their employees or provide classes on appropriate patient guidance, but again, some regulations miss the mark. For example, in Connecticut, dispensary owners must be certified pharmacists. This is a good attempt at medical standardization, but since pharmacists do not study cannabis in pharmacy school, their knowledge may be considerably less than that of your average philosophy major who smoked regularly in college.

Rules for caregivers (friends or family members who apply to provide marijuana to patients) are also prevalent in the current laws in many states. In Colorado, caregivers may serve no more than five patients. In Massachusetts, caregivers are limited to one patient. In California, caregivers must prove that they provide care for the patient, but once again, they are not required to have any specific knowledge about cannabis.

These caregivers often grow the patient's marijuana as well. Defining rules for gardening a weed that can be as small as a seedling or as large as a hedge is difficult. Proposition 215, with one of the more rational approaches to growing—because it was based on number of square feet, not plant numbers—allowed caregivers to grow five hundred square feet of cannabis if they had fewer than five patients. (If my five hundred-square-foot operation was serving two hundred patients, then five patients in California must consume a lot of marijuana.) Currently in Massachusetts, residents over twenty-one can now grow up to twelve plants per household, with no specified square footage limit. Thus, if a plant grows to be over seven feet by seven feet in area, then those twelve plants will exceed five hundred square feet of space, providing far in excess of the possession limit of ten ounces every sixty days.

None of the growing rules take into account the varying concentrations of THC in the plant. Some strains can have 15 percent THC in their flowers, and some can have 30 percent. In an attempt to address this confusion, some states, like Connecticut, still do not allow home cultivation. The irony in this case is that a patient can bring home cannabis from a legal dispensary and *accidentally* become a criminal if a seed from the cannabis inadvertently drops into the home garden patch and germinates. Unlike opium, cocaine, and other plant-based drugs, the marijuana plant requires almost no processing (other than the summer growth cycle) to produce the potent active ingredient. It is interesting to note that the common poppy, flowering in gardens everywhere, is responsible for the resin that produces methadone and ultimately heroin. For some reason, poppies, as well as *Nocotiana tabacum,* another flowering ornamental also known as the highly carcinogenic tobacco plant, are not ripped out of gardens by DEA agents.

Although not a single state requires specific knowledge of cannabis or the endocannabinoid system in their medical or recreational marijuana regulations, Proposition 215 was not completely devoid of medical context. It did require the development of a medical marijuana research program in the California university system using "state-of-the-art research methodologies."[43] This was in part due to the fact that several years earlier, a group of Israeli researchers, led by Raphael Mechoulam, synthesized and named the endogenous chemical anandamide. The class of chemicals anandamide uncovered, which are naturally produced in essentially every animal species on Earth except for insects, was named from the Sanskrit word for "bliss." Anandamide was discovered by tracing the action of exogenous or plant-made phytocannabinoids in the body.[44] It seemed that the active phytocannabinoid, tetrahydrocannabinol (THC) in cannabis mimicked anandamide and fit into these previously unknown anandamide receptor sites like keys entering a lock. Thus, the newly discovered internal feedback system was named *endo,* meaning "in," and *cannabinoid,* meaning compounds similar to those found in cannabis. Today, scientists all over the world are conducting research on the endocannabinoid system (ECS). One does not have to involve the cannabis plant to perform the research, but the loaded word "canna" in the name probably doesn't help doctors open up to the vast medical implications of this feedback system.

Some doctors have come around to appreciate the medicinal benefits of cannabis, but many lack any medical knowledge on the subject. In their defense, doctors often have to avoid anything cannabis related because their careers are dependent on appearing conservative and sober. They also have little access to the subject in medical school. In a 2014 survey of every accredited medical school in the United States, only 13 percent of institutions even mentioned the endocannabinoid system in their courses.[45] Dr. David Allen, a cannabis researcher who conducted the survey, reflects on the results:

> There is no reason our potential medical doctors should be ignorant of this important physiologic control mechanism. This is similar to ignoring a medical field like neuroanatomy. The majority of people in the United States have no idea of the remarkable, scientifically proven medical benefits of cannabis. These cannabinoids are responsible for massive reductions in diabetes [and] stroke. Many cancers show significant responses to cannabinoids. Glucose and fatty metabolism, pain control and inflammation are all controlled by the ECS. There are many reports of patients with seizures that are unresponsive to all medicines except cannabis extracts. We are learning that even the sperm implantation into the ovum requires endocannabinoids for success. Mother's milk contains endocannabinoids that stimulate the infant to feed and thrive. (This transfer of cannabinoids from mother to child is the only still [federally] legal transfer of exogenous cannabinoids).[46]

Over a decade after medical marijuana was legalized in California, Dr. Donald Abrams, another doctor who has conducted much research on the subject, including successful cannabis trials for AIDS patients in California, declared, "I don't think anybody bothers to really look at the research being done or make any policy changes on the basis of it."[47] The neurologist Dr. Ethan Russo, who has spent decades compiling much of the clinical and historical evidence regarding cannabis, summarizes the medical evidence from India alone: "The vast majority of claims for cannabis from India are fully corroborated by modern scientific and clinical investigation."[48]

So what gives? Despite the fact that medical evidence exists and the "state of the art methodologies" were passed in California over twenty years ago, we still have little consistent data about what a proper dose is, what strains work for what ailments, and how an individual will respond to a specific ingestion method. We have hundreds of studies detailing the medicinal effects of cannabinoids, from collecting medical data on patients who smoke regularly to analyzing human cells that are bathed in cannabinoids in a petri dish to genetically engineering mice to have active or inactive endocannabinoid systems. We now know it works, but we can't necessarily create a perfect little pill that will have the same effect over and over. When it comes to treating individuals successfully, a common refrain used by practitioners and retail clerks alike is still, "Start low and go slow." Often, patients can know what works only by trial and error or by titrating up over time in order to see how it is affecting symptoms. The difficulty of creating a standard pill or dose is in part due to the fact that cannabis works better in whole-plant form. It has been discovered that isolated cannabinoid molecules working alone do not have as strong an effect as the whole plant's molecules working together. This is now referred to as the "entourage effect."[49] And because we each have a unique endocannabinoid system ebbing and flowing in its diverse action all over our body, it's difficult to predict which combination of cannabinoids at which amount will have the desired effect. The effect on an individual can also change and evolve over time, as anyone knows who smoked happily in college but now feels that cannabis just makes him paranoid.

This discrepancy is not a bad thing. It just means that cannabis does not fit into an FDA-approved drug model that requires each molecule in a pill to be exact and replicable. The entourage effect exists in an area of medicine that is neither conventional nor purely herbal. Most herbs do not cause a powerful psychoactive response, let alone regulate an intrinsic system that affects almost every cell in our body. Cannabis exists in the middle ground: a powerful medicine, easily grown at home, that is nontoxic but extremely powerful in its ability to regulate disease as well as alter consciousness.

Medicinal or recreational marijuana use is now legal in a majority of states in the United States. Eventually, the federal government and other countries will follow. Although the laws controlling it ebb and flow, cannabis in all its forms has been grown continually in the United States for over four hundred years. It is growing in the wild, and your spouse or teenager may be secretly growing it in a closet in your home. It is here to stay. The context we bring to this ubiquitous and controversial plant will influence how it is used by adults and children. If laws eventually allow pot shops to function like liquor stores, with bud tenders selling to whoever comes in and presents an ID, then *medical* marijuana may be a windy road of trial and error for the patients who could benefit from it. Some will take more and more THC to combat their symptoms, not realizing that a more holistic approach to the diverse array of cannabinoids is needed. Many users in this scenario will succumb to its addictive nature. The effect will still be a net benefit to the community in comparison to opioid addiction, which kills thousands of Americans every year. But I believe it is the role of the cannabis dispensary, the community, of families, practitioners, caregivers, friends, and spouses to have forthright conversations with users. Out of empathy, they need to understand and monitor the use of a person's cannabis in order to ensure that it is contributing to sustained and improved health. A bud tender or even a doctor who sees dozens of medical marijuana clients a day may miss that a patient needs to take a break from cannabis. They may not be able to see that same patient again when he or she comes in with more questions. A patient who continues to smoke pot for anxiety, for example, may actually be exacerbating the ailment, and the vicious cycle of abuse is missed by the patient's doctor or favorite bud tender.

Although we now have schools and courses training bud tenders how to advise patients, and the culture of many dispensaries is one of compassion and medicinal focus, there is no standard for guidance because there is no standard for a whole-plant drug with a myriad of forms. What works to help a bud tender sleep may make a customer toss and turn all night long. Many patients who seek a more natural treatment for their ailments will want to build trust with the person providing the cannabis and will want to have access to that same individual when they have questions. Their doctor may support using it, but many patients feel confused and uncomfortable walking into a dispensary outfitted with more surveillance cameras than educational pamphlets. Others may want the relaxed, legal setting of a dispensary, with the knowledge and privacy of their health practitioner's office. We also have segments of the population that privately benefit from cannabis, but due to their standing in the community as health providers or government workers, they cannot publicly wait in line at a dispensary to procure cannabis, for fear of being exposed. They may instead get their marijuana illegally from friends or "dealers," but the culture of acquiring marijuana from a private source is not necessarily a nefarious one. Many public employees, lawyers, teachers, and doctors still break the law to acquire cannabis, in order to maintain their privacy and keep their ailments at bay. Many of these upstanding citizens were my clients.

Because I empathize with the people facing these dilemmas, I hope the stories and conversations in this book can serve as a model for how patients, practitioners, and caregivers can know when and how to use cannabis and when to back off and take a break. Parents should learn how to talk to their children before abuse sets in. And those who will never set foot in a dispensary will know how to start their own medicinal garden in their home.

Now that we have thousands of dispensaries serving millions of patients, and marijuana laws relaxing across the country, with defendants like myself setting a new legal precedent, I believe we should encourage a diverse cannabis culture that is informed, that expresses empathy for patients, and that respects the power of this plant to harm and to heal. Cannabis practitioners with a small basement garden in their home could easily and safely serve a roster of fifty clients. The idea that we might legalize a home grower's selling of medical marijuana to his or her community may sound shocking to some, but it is already being done safely all over the world. Growers who provide remedies to their community are hidden underground because law enforcement can arrest them, seize their assets, put their children in foster care, and send them to federal prison—all while the local dispensary can legally churn out thousands of pounds of cannabis to users who may be abusing the drug, using it to their detriment, or selling it to minors. Communities that are informed about this disparity will be better placed to create sensible regulation.

Mixed Messages

A simple starting point for how to use cannabis as medicine is to put it in context with the health and regulatory model of medicines we already utilize. The most obvious health practitioner we might seek out to answer medical marijuana questions might be a family doctor or psychologist. Surely they know whether cannabis is dangerous and what its effects are on the children who might already watch family members consume it legally. Do the legislatures writing the regulations for this politically charged plant know the difference between a stoner "just getting high" and a patient weaning him- or herself off opioids or managing a debilitating disease with multiple forms of cannabis? The famous stoners of the world, like Cheech and Chong, or advocates like Woody Harrelson or Willie Nelson think that smoking pot is no big deal. For them it's okay. (The majority of adults in America now agree.[50]) But do these provocateurs have children? Why are some doctors prescribing it to children, while others are dismissing their actions as irresponsible quackery or worse? Who do we ask to interpret the facts and the real science on the subject?

It is likely that many medical schools do not have courses or whole departments devoted to the human body's ECS because the research is relatively recent and it has not seemed relevant up to now. If the federal government were to reschedule cannabis from Schedule I, a dangerous drug with no medical benefits, to a drug like cocaine, methamphetamine, or methadone (all Schedule II drugs), more medical schools and research universities could study it. Cannabis research has had its own difficulties with perception and the influence of entities in the government, such as the National Institute of Drug Abuse (NIDA). NIDA, owing to the Drug Enforcement Administration's mandate designed to prevent the diversion of marijuana, requires all researchers to obtain marijuana from a single source: the substandard cannabis production facility at the University of Mississippi. Whereas researchers studying cocaine can access medical-grade product, the growers in Mississippi are not incentivized (or allowed?) to grow the high-end cannabis that is readily available to illicit and legal consumers. Thus, scientists who are trying to understand the medicinal effects of cannabis already being consumed all over the country can wait years to study plant material that is capable of medicating few. But despite NIDA's oppressive rules for research, the Brookings Institute, in their 2015 report *Ending the U.S. Government's War on Medical Marijuana Research,* states, "Rescheduling will not suddenly legalize marijuana. It would not even solve the policy disjunction that exists between states and the federal government on the question of marijuana legality—or even [medicinal] value. Nor does rescheduling mean that medical marijuana will line the shelves of commercial or hospital pharmacies."[51] So this will be a problem for legislatures and the FDA for years to come.

But in my opinion, there is enough evidence already out there to allow patients to try it. It's not a laboratory-made molecule. A person who grows marijuana and feels the positive effects on his symptoms has all the evidence he needs. Medically, cannabis is far-reaching in its positive effects.

Regardless of federal regulation and scheduling status, roughly twenty-two million people still use cannabis in the United States on a daily basis.[52] More research will eventually occur, but bona fide, double-blind experiments have already shown the ability of cannabis to ease nausea more effectively than do some conventional antiemetic drugs.[53] It's been proven effective for pain and appetite stimulation, literally extending the lives of cancer and AIDS patients who suffer from wasting syndrome and can't eat.[54] These are not obscure studies. These are controlled studies published by the U.S. National Institutes of Health (NIH). The National Cancer Institute categorizes on its Web site all the animal and human trials attesting to its anti-tumor, antiemetic, and analgesic effects, as well as its effectiveness for inducing sleep and in reducing anxiety.[55]

The DEA administrators are mandating cannabis's Schedule I status—that it is a dangerous drug with no medical uses—because of cultural *perception*, mainly theirs. In the DEA's own seventy-page position on marijuana, published in 2013, they cite the stance of several health organizations, including the American Medical Association, the American Cancer Society, and the American Institute of Medicine.[56] The DEA confirms that they all agree there may be benefits to using cannabis medically. The health organizations state that more research is needed (but are careful to articulate that they do not advocate the legalization of marijuana). The DEA sums up its response to their measured yet curious stance on the drug with the statement, "Smoked marijuana is not medicine." It seems like common sense and may sound good to parents and those ignorant of the drug, but it is akin to saying, "Smoked ibuprofen is not medicine." The DEA also has the power to influence statements and opinions regarding cannabis, because its agents enforce the law. They are the ones funding the military helicopters that patrol suburban backyards in legal and illegal states, looking for cannabis. If you're an established health organization and you state that you think cannabis is a promising medicine, you are directly contradicting the DEA and the law of the land. Your statement could be interpreted as conspiring to break the law. It's like announcing to the state police officers that you believe some speeds in excess of the posted limit are safe for travel. They then have the power to make your life very difficult. Because of your statement, they have probable cause to follow you around everywhere you drive. Thus, few health professionals, let alone whole health organizations, have the guts to contradict the DEA (except the aforementioned NIH and the National Cancer Institute, paradoxically).

Although the DEA has a stranglehold on cannabis research, the drugs that do pass the FDA's strict requirements are not necessarily harmless. It is common knowledge that prescription opioids are more dangerous than any form of cannabis, smoked or otherwise. Legal prescription opioids killed more people between 1999 and 2008 than cocaine and heroin overdoses combined.[57] There are also dozens of FDA-approved drugs that have been taken *off* the market because of the harm they later caused.[58]

Numerous plants are the basis for synthetic drugs, and thousands of drugs exist. But adding to the uphill battle, whole plants making it onto the *United States Pharmacopeia* are incredibly rare. Whole plants present too many variables for them to be patented or studied effectively.[59] They may be effective, but they don't fit nicely into the structure of the FDA approval process, just as one-of-a-kind, handcrafted widgets are hard to find at a box store chain. If a researcher is conducting a drug trial, the molecule in question has to be consistent and discrete.

We take comfort in knowing that a drug researcher in a white coat worked tirelessly to develop a little pill in a sophisticated lab. This is the new era where powerful pills outstrip the plodding evolution of nature or an apothecary's handmade remedy. Technological progress prevails. Thus, pharmaceutical companies have an easy in with overworked doctors. Pharmaceutical representatives are paid to convince doctors to use their FDA-approved drugs. The companies do all the research and development, the FDA makes sure the drugs are safe, and the doctor just has to scribble a prescription on a piece of paper. Voilà—we all benefit from the wonders of modern medical science. For millions of Americans, the benefits are real. Swallowing the pill *can* make our problems go away. The system grows toward this ideal, but many individual patients suffer within it. Large-scale trials that determine a drug's effectiveness, even if they are 80 percent successful, still leave 20 percent of patients with no positive results, or even negative responses to drugs years later. The system is not perfect. Over three-quarters of trials in the United States are funded by drug companies themselves.[60] Pharmaceutical companies have their shareholders to please, after all. If patients take fewer drugs, the business model suffers. So we take these drugs that are directly responsible for half a million deaths in the West every year.[61] Based on an FDA report, each year there are over a million serious cases of adverse drug reactions in the United States, leading to thousands of lives lost.[62] Patients need options, but selling more of these drugs does not automatically mean more lives will be saved. The upshot is that the federal government is sending mixed messages about drugs and about cannabis. It is a disaster for the hundreds of thousands of marijuana arrestees around the country every year. It confuses parents and erodes children's trust in the drug pamphlets they see at school. And it is a tragedy for the millions of suffering patients who could benefit from a scientifically efficacious, nonfatal medicine.

This notion of basing decisions on perception instead of data is not unheard of. Humans are not a rational species, and society and culture frequently exist in gray areas. Whole fields of study, such as philosophy and history, rest in gray areas of nuance and subjectivity. Airplanes are the safest method of travel, but turbulence and the specter of terrorism make air travel terrifying for many. Thus, we are comforted by terms like "precision medicine" and "top ten hospitals in the country," but disease and its treatment can be messy and organic. One person's positive response to a therapy, surgery, or medication can be another's malpractice suit.

Many doctors and researchers want to believe that health processes are not organic, that the body's physiological ailments can be addressed regardless of the patients' perception of treatment. But for many symptoms, it is not that simple. As Dr. Jo Marchant writes in *Cure: The Journey into the Science of Mind over Body*, "Psychological factors such as stress can trigger the release of neurotransmitters that influence immune responses, while chemicals released by the immune system can in turn influence the brain."[63] We are more than the sum total of the parts in our body. Our mind, spirit, faith, and opinions, and our relationship with those who care for us, all contribute to our well-being. Subjective perception plays a role in medicine. To add to this complexity, cannabis alters our perception.

One of the most controversial aspects of marijuana is that it may be hurting our brains as it opens us up to different facets of perception. But a study conducted by the *Journal of Alzheimer's Disease* concluded that it didn't hurt Alzheimer's patients' brains; instead, it found that "adding medical cannabis oil to Alzheimer's patients' pharmacotherapy is a safe and promising treatment option."[64] As I dug into the scientific or historical evidence of its medical efficacy, the refrain began to shine through: marijuana's spectrum of medical efficacy is vast. Yet it is still considered a drug with no medical benefits. Perhaps its healing attributes, to doctors, just sound too good to be true. For example, how can a drug that helps with neuropathic pain[65] also relieve anxiety[66] *and* detoxify the liver after cocaine toxicity?[67] How could a sophisticated pharmaceutical, let alone an illicit drug smoked by college students and urban youth, possibly come close to addressing so many ailments? Scientifically speaking, the answer is complex and may never be categorically solved. But in layman's terms, the answer is simple. Cannabinoids serve as regulators in trillions of cells in the body. Like traffic lights managing traffic buildup at an intersection, cannabinoids are released and received by cells to keep homeostasis intact in the cell and thus the organism. Cannabinoids' role is to act on cells in the nervous and immune system, in order to bring them back to their baseline behavior. These cells are connected with every organ, bone, muscle, and nerve in our body. Cannabinoids have such a broad effect on body and mind (and perhaps consciousness) because they interact with the two systems in the body researchers used to think were separate.

A psychologist named Dr. Bob Ader discovered in the 1970s that not only are the immune and nervous systems connected physiologically, but their relationship has alarming results. He performed an experiment on mice, giving them sugar water infused with a chemical that made them feel sick by suppressing their immune systems. He was training the mice to associate sugar water with sickness. He later wanted to see how long it took them to forget the association by force-feeding them plain sugar water. Instead of changing their association with the sugar water over time, their nervous systems collapsed and the mice succumbed to fatal infection.[68] We might say it was their nervous system's *belief* that they were dying that caused the physiological reality. Later experiments backed up this bizarre result with observations of nerves running through nervous system organs such as the spleen and thymus.[69] There is an inextricable connection between our nervous system—how we experience the world—and our immune system that protects us from it.

Our internal or "endo" cannabinoids as well as external or "phyto" cannabinoids do their dance where these two systems meet. And cannabinoids make us *feel* a certain way. Anandamide, the endocannabinoid we produce that is mimicked by THC, is thought to give us the "runner's high" after we exercise.[70] For years, the consensus has been that we have two main cell receptor sites for receiving cannabinoids. As of this writing, there is speculation that a third may be present, because sometimes cannabinoids affect cell behavior without interacting with the CB1 or CB2 receptor sites.[71] The science is new and unfolding. Individual stories of patients help clarify the wide spectrum of potential response, because clinical trials have difficulty accounting for every variable and every perception of the patient. For example, some users report an intolerable response to marijuana and others feel nothing at all. It is not yet known precisely why this is the case. I have had clients try the same oil that had elicited a profoundly divergent response. In the course of a week, one client told me she tried three drops (less than 3 mg of THC), which she said felt "like taking an entire bottle of speed." She couldn't sleep all night, owing to the extremity of the reaction. The other client called me up to complain, as she had gone through an entire bottle (approximately 250 mg of THC) of the same oil over the course of twenty-four hours. Because she felt no response whatsoever, she questioned whether I was trying to rip her off and wanted her money back.

Thus, instead of merely having clinical evidence for how cannabis can help patients, what may help is to recontextualize cannabis. If the theory is true of the nervous and immune systems being inextricably connected, recontextualization may be important to the body's reception of cannabis. We have to accept how our body and mind respond, not only to the drug but to the setting in which it was given. Did we feel heard by the doctor or bud tender? Are we in agreement with our caretaker and spouse about the treatment protocol? These questions effect the attitude and morale of the patient. I tell my clients that our belly is filled with trillions of neurons and that some researchers consider it our "second brain."[72] If we have a negative gut feeling about a drug or the person writing a prescription for it, then changing that gut feeling to positive could cause a healthier response.

In order to change cultural perception about anything from Copernican theory to climate change, more nuance is needed than raw science. I can also appreciate that many patients or caregivers aren't ready to experiment with non–FDA-verified drugs. But I do find it strange that we don't even have a different name for "drugs" sold at drugstores and "drugs" sold on the street by drug dealers. When kids hear "Say no to drugs," who determines which drugs they should say no to? Apparently we're to say yes to FDA-approved drugs and no to drugs like cannabis. Thus, I might suggest that a patient try a specific remedy, but because I don't have a medical degree, and cannabis is still considered a substance with no medical benefits, I also work hard to make my clients' *experience* as comfortable as possible. I want them to leave with the knowledge that they were heard and received empathy and that when the remedy has differing results or doesn't work, I'll be there to explain and puzzle out what happened.

When the health care system is so cumbersome that a third of all deaths are caused by medical error,[73] then we might ask ourselves this question: How can we as individuals help reduce pressure on that system? Cannabis is not a magic bullet, but like healthy vegetables grown at home, it also does not require FDA approval, large-scale clinical trials, or doctors to prescribe it for benefits to be felt. Dr. Casserett, the author of *Stoned: A Physician's Case for Medical Marijuana,* found that the patients he talked to "weren't turning to medical marijuana [solely] because of its benefits, but because it gave them control of their ailments. It let them manage their health in a way that was productive, effective, and comfortable for them."[74] Even a recreational dispensary that does not purport to provide *medical* marijuana may still offer comfort and camaraderie to a patient who feels disempowered by the sterile environs of for-profit hospitals or bustling doctors' offices. Once a patient does develop a relationship with a dispensary or caregiver, he or she can begin to access the control Dr. Casserett witnessed. But the magic of cannabis is that individuals can alter their own health or that of their loved ones with this powerful herb all by themselves. Taking into account its ancient medicinal history and its effect on our nervous and immune systems, we can turn to homegrown cannabis as providing another option for addressing bodily ailments as well as the disempowerment many patients experience in dealing with the medical system.

Medical Marijuana Patient or Drug Addict?

When medical marijuana was legalized in the state of Massachusetts, I had already been growing cannabis illegally for a couple of years, but being a veteran science and art teacher with a master's degree, I wondered if I could bring a measure of professionalism and intellect to the field as it took root in my community. Suffering from teacher burnout and with much hand-wringing about the unpredictability of a pot career, I took the leap and quit my teaching job. Disappointingly, no dispensaries would open for more than two years after the law passed, so I scrambled to find a job working at a garden store that specialized in "hydroponics," a euphemism for indoor marijuana cultivation. I wanted to know as much about growing and the field as I could, so I figured it was a good place to start. It was also where I met my first medical marijuana patients and began to develop my approach to helping people access cannabis medicinally.

One morning, I sat behind the counter of the small garden shop eating a sandwich when a large, limping man came in and introduced himself as Johnny. He was in his fifties, overweight, and boisterous. His white hair was rebelling against an earlier comb. He wore a dark blue golf shirt that rucked up around his left side, where his elbow was held in a complicated steel brace. I could see multiple scars meandering up his left arm, where a wool mitten covered his hand.

Johnny was in pain and he was pissed. An old foot injury hindered his gait and contributed to his obesity. A year earlier, after falling through a broken railing while limping up a wheelchair ramp, his left arm had sustained nerve damage and become paralyzed. Despite a dozen surgeries, his pain was worse than ever. Some of the surgeries had helped, some had failed. Some of the surgeons had made mistakes. Along with pills, he drank the edge off the pain, until alcoholism caused more damage to his life, so he quit drinking. Now the pain was constant. Countless opioids and other medications coursed through his body, wreaking havoc on his liver, his GI tract, his sleep cycle, and his normally jovial mood.

After using marijuana casually in his youth, he rediscovered it after his fall forced him into early retirement from managing a car dealership. He wanted to keep working, but the pain was too severe. Once the medical marijuana law passed, he got his state-licensed card and was determined to produce as much medical marijuana as he could. He gathered a team to open a dispensary. Although they had the capital, they had not passed the first round of dispensary applications. They had spent months on filing proper paperwork to the state. Despite their not making it to the second round, for "unspecified reasons," the state had kept their $35,000 application fee.

He leaned in to speak to me, his head cocked to one side—out of pain, or just piss and vinegar, I couldn't tell.

"I don't give a fuck. I'm going to sue the guy who fucked up my arm. I'm going to sue the surgeons who fucked it up worse. I'm going to sue the state for their bullshit dispensary rules and my $35,000. And now I'm going to start a garden. I'm going to put it on my credit card, and you're going to help me do it," he said, smacking his card on the table. When a person uses plastic and not cash in a marijuana grow store, you know he's tired of hiding.

"Actually, I've been thinking about offering consultations to people starting their gardens. I could come take a look at your space after work if you want," I offered. The grow store was not paying enough to cover my bills. My little basement garden was a source of illegal income from friends, but I felt I could offer a wider range of legal services through consultation. I hadn't scratched the surface of medical marijuana beyond my evening stress relief, but I figured I could help clients grow their own, since it was legal for patients to grow a limited amount for their own consumption.

Johnny was comfortable enough with marijuana to know that it was helping his ailments, but he didn't know where to get it in the quantities he needed. When he had enough marijuana, he was able to reduce his meds significantly. He now smoked a lot, as I could smell when he came into the store. I told him I'd stop by that evening.

Johnny's lifestyle seemed to fulfill the stoner stereotype I was trying to avoid as a cannabis professional. His house was cluttered in every corner.

Spilled cat dishes littered coffee tables. A big, worn-out recliner in the living room sat surrounded by tray tables filled with pill bottles, smoking paraphernalia, and legal paperwork. Scrambling to get their grow going, he and his wife had cleared out two bedrooms, their contents piled up in the dining room. His house was in disarray, but his garden was coming along nicely. Entering his grow area was like entering a manicured botanical garden. The plants were well maintained, water and HVAC systems efficient, floors swept. The work to acquire effective medicine had inspired a level of meticulousness not applied to other aspects of his life. And with two bedrooms serving as his garden, he could easily grow a couple of pounds a month. His wife was a civil engineer for the state and came home every night to take the edge off her knee pain and smoke with Johnny. She had had a couple of unsuccessful knee surgeries herself.

I came back several times over the months to get him and his wife up and running. He called me after harvest time and we toured his new set of crops before he grew achy and needed to settle back into his recliner.

"I'm doing good, right Ezra? Right!?" He asked as he unscrewed gallon-sized mason jars and made several small piles of marijuana flower buds on a TV tray.

"You're doing great, Johnny. Those plants are beautiful. The buds are enormous. Temperatures are stable. You're doing really well!" I replied. I would rather have gotten back to my family after a long workday, but apparently among pot smokers, visiting fellow enthusiasts without sharing a puff is almost a sacrilege. It's a part of the culture that I have never felt comfortable with. I prefer to partake after work in the privacy of my own home. Although cannabis is my profession, I am not able to work while high. But I was new to the field, so figured I would acclimate to the culture as best I could. He handed me a grinder and I set out to pulverize the cured buds with my two good hands.

He talked while he worked the enormous jars. "Oh my God, did you smell that one? It smells so fucking good. This one is my favorite. It gets me ripped, but it also takes the pain away. Here—grind these up, too, will ya? I want you to taste all these. I have the best fucking bud, Ezra! I'll get the vape warmed up! I'm doing good, right buddy!?" His eyes widened as he sought my approval.

"You are doing good, Johnny. The garden is beautiful." It was dawning on me what the plan was with all of the ground-up marijuana piles on Johnny's TV tray. He was going to warm up his tabletop vaporizing machine, a toaster-sized metal box with a digital readout and a long tube coming out of it. We were going to "taste" each of his newly cured strains. By my count, the piles on the tray amounted to enough marijuana for a couple of people to get high continually for at least a week. It equaled roughly thirty joints.

"Finally, I can medicate with my own medicine! And look, I can move my fingers!" He pulled the mitten off his pale and swollen left hand, revealing shiny incision scars along each finger. They trembled as he tried to bend them. "Ah fuck. It fucking hurts. I'm still going to sue the motherfuckers, but at least I'm not drinking. That's huge. Drinking really messed up my life. And I've cut my opioids down by 90 percent. Can you believe that? I don't have to go to the doctor or pharmacy every week. That alone makes me feel better. That's why I want to celebrate! I want you to try my first harvest."

"That is amazing, Johnny. Congrats," I said. "Though you realize that after I try the first pile, I will have no ability to 'taste' or distinguish it from the other seven samples on the tray." I was and still am a lightweight when it comes to smoking cannabis. Johnny was a living example of the blurry line between medical and recreational cannabis because he loved it, consumed as much as humanly possible, and he seemed to benefit from it medically.

"Dude. I'm just proud of myself. I just want you to try all my strains. Ahh, my arm fucking hurts. I want you to try what you helped me grow. You're my best friend!" He finished loading the huge vape chamber one-handed, and after the light turned green on the toaster, he drew an enormous breath from the tube. His cheeks reddened and sweat dripped down his face from the pain. It might have been tears. I couldn't tell.

I wasn't really his best friend, and I knew he was a serious marijuana addict, but we both knew he was happy he wasn't addicted to alcohol or opioids anymore. He'd lost a few pounds over the months, and although he was as foulmouthed as ever, Johnny was every day more joyful about his self-sustaining garden. It made him happy and gave him purpose. Hauling water and plants around his garden rooms kept his body moving. He started buying more vegetables from local farmer's markets, as well.

Johnny's wide frame stretched out his pink polo shirt as he inhaled a breath from the tube and passed it to me. I would have gotten plenty stoned with his second-hand smoke. When he exhaled, Johnny gulped and sniffed at the smoke curling from his lips. To the untrained eye, he was a chronic user, someone who was probably high twenty-four hours a day. His cluttered lifestyle flushed out a stereotype of a pothead who couldn't get off the couch and clean his house. But he was also a medical user who would be destitute without cannabis. He did get off his couch—painfully—to water his plants and keep his garden producing because the plant renewed his hope and health.

Few people fall in love with their pharmaceuticals. It's partly why we have a hard time with medical marijuana as a culture. If we love it so much, then is it really a medicine? Aren't people who love their drug just drug addicts? For Johnny, it was his medicine and his life. And it is not a judgment question that can be answered on a large scale. The experience is subjective. Cannabis growing provides users with the ultimate freedom to decide whether they want to succumb to a stereotype or increase the quality of their lives. Without access to cannabis, Johnny's high tolerance for drugs may have made him a victim of opioid overdose. He consumes a full ounce of cannabis every thirty-six hours. He also goes bird-watching on the weekends, eats well, and has a fulfilling marriage.

His wife came home and joined us downstairs with a chuckle. "Ezra must have smoked that CBD strain. He's lilting." I righted myself from the forty-five-degree angle I had leaned into on the couch. I tried to take deep, measured breaths to keep the waves of pot-induced anxiety at bay. Johnny laughed, his pained expression replaced with glassy-eyed joy.

After witnessing Johnny's medical transformation, I started to hit the scholarly articles to figure out what cannabis was actually doing for symptoms and diseases. I found studies showing the cannabinoids and the endocannabinoid system regulated the immune system,[75] mitigated neurological disorders,[76] fought cancer cells,[77] and reduced inflammation.[78] The symptoms of diseases such as Parkinson's,[79] arthritis,[80] and fibromyalgia[81] were reduced in clinical studies on cannabinoids. When I typed the words "cannabinoid" and "scholarly" into a search engine, I found that researchers had done countless studies on cannabis and cannabinoids. I admit it was shocking to discover that a plant known for making people slaphappy also regulated the very unhappy Crohn's disease.[82]

If cannabinoids showed promise in treating pain in clinical trials, then why weren't practitioners rallying around it to help their patients? Was it because people like Johnny, although helped medically, gave it a bad name? I met a grower at the garden shop who brought his medical marijuana card to his primary physician and asked her what she thought about his using marijuana successfully for his back pain instead of opioids. She dismissed his comment as hearsay and wrote on his report: "Patient abuses illegal drugs." This statement would be in his medical records for life. I called up the head of the teaching wing of my local hospital and asked him if he and his colleagues had looked into its possibilities for symptom reduction based on the studies. "I know there are medical benefits, but the vast majority of users are just trying to get high. They should just legalize it like alcohol and be done with it," he said. I wondered if his response summed up an ethos in the medical community surrounding cannabis that I began to fear might prevail if we don't seek to understand its medicinal uses: that it is a drug purely for escape and recreational purposes. Its subtle medicinal properties could be lost in the thick smoke of recreational use, as laws and communities become more relaxed about its use.

His answer only inspired me to dig deeper. I read hundreds of studies easily accessible on legitimate scholarly Web sites, such as PubMed and Google Scholar. I had uncovered a gold mine of medical data. Perhaps nobody trusted the glassy-eyed believers who linked to these studies on their pot-leaf-adorned Web sites. A study of a compound's effect on a patient requires additional studies to confirm that it is safe. But people smoked cannabis and ate pot brownies all over the world. They grew it in their homes. It wasn't a laboratory-made chemical. I, with my degree in art, had been creating this pharmaceutical for years. People like Johnny were total stoners, but they were medical marijuana patients as well. If cannabis wasn't killing Johnny and his wife the way opioids could, then even his chronic addiction to pot was a net benefit to his life, in my opinion. In any community, this would equal fewer pills, fewer hospital visits, and fewer overdoses. In a country where opioid overdose kills close to a hundred people a day,[83] informed cannabis use became a cause worth fighting for.

There was nothing illegal about sharing ideas and education with medical marijuana patients. I realized I was sober and professional enough to bring my skills to other patients like Johnny. If I saw them in my own home, then I wouldn't have to smoke with them. My basement garden was stable and consistent. Since I didn't derive a lot of benefit from smoking socially, I mainly focused on developing remedies and getting people well. I also made contact with a couple of doctors in the area who needed someone to whom they could send their patients for advice. Within a year, I had two employees working with me full-time. I provided plants and medical cannabis remedies to over two hundred patients, with ailments as diverse as regional pain syndrome and PTSD.

Out of the Closet

I took my newfound research and became an outspoken cannabis educator in the community. Although I was skirting the law, I felt that hiding in the shadows perpetuated stereotypes of cannabis as illicit. When people were suffering and dying from so many of the diseases that cannabis was effective at treating, the idea that it was illicit became anathema to me. I became as frustrated with the medical community as with the culture that perpetuated its lowbrow recreational use. News articles reporting on its medical benefits found in a laboratory study would still show an unrelated image of a person smoking a joint. As I was beginning to see clients who had lost control of their health and wanted to try marijuana only as a last resort, the stereotypical images made me cringe. I wanted to help change cultural perceptions. When three local news outlets joined forces to host a panel on the subject, they asked if I would participate. Despite the legal risk of further exposure, I jumped at the chance. They wanted to have a medical marijuana patient on the panel as well, so I reached out to my clients for volunteers.

The war on drugs in America has been carried on for generations, leaving many adults deeply fearful of revealing their cannabis use or support of the drug. People often wonder why I was so open about my profession and allowed unknown clients to come to my home where I grew cannabis. One could say I had "white privilege" and didn't understand the risks of getting caught. This is true. I had never been arrested and had never been pulled over by a police officer, unless I was actually breaking a traffic law. Perhaps I trusted police officers' humanness and figured they'd let me go when they saw how upstanding I was. But the white privilege argument only goes so far. Naïveté did not drive my actions—justice did. I empathized with people like Johnny, and I also spent a decade teaching in impoverished black and Latino communities that felt the tangible effects from the drug war. I had students with cannabis tattoos on their arms. They weren't fearful of police action, but they deserved to be. Many cannabis smokers might be using it for purely recreational reasons, but even that line is blurry. I believe taking a substance that helps you better participate in your adult life is a personal right. Marijuana was prevalent in my students' lives, but because of the poverty in which they lived, on average they would die earlier, have more physical disability, higher rates of asthma, and experience more clinical depression throughout their lives.[84] I once asked a visiting social worker how many of the students she thought might suffer from PTSD. "A hundred percent," she answered without hesitation. Perhaps they, too, were seeking a mixture of its medical and recreational benefits.

I understood intuitively why my students might gravitate toward cannabis. Their lives were often traumatic. But I later found out that my intuition was backed up by science. Research suggests the cannabinoids in the weed they smoked might be helping mitigate trauma by distancing them from memories of the event.[85] Many of us worry that pot will make us forgetful. Perhaps many teenagers are subconsciously using it *for* this purpose. The endocannabinoid system is also thought to be connected to neurons associated with stress reduction.[86] Ingesting cannabis for stress relief isn't something a teacher should shun as irresponsible. I thought about the inner-city neighborhoods across the nation filled with kids like my students: impoverished, disenfranchised, and underrepresented teens who gravitated toward cannabis or were surrounded by people who self-medicated with it. I had many students who suffered from trauma, asthma, and anxiety who were also using marijuana. It is not intuitive, but smoked cannabis has been shown to reduce asthma symptoms in a placebo-controlled study.[87] But if they get caught smoking pot, the punishment and disruption to their lives may exacerbate their stress-related ailments, and the cycle continues.

I was not as out of the closet about pot as some of my students were, but as a middle-class white man with a decade of connection to students of color, I felt a sense of duty to correct the public stance on the drug in the hope that fewer arrests would be made in my students' communities. I wanted to raise a fist in protest, but I didn't feel comfortable smoking pot at a public rally or holding "legalize it" picket signs. Consuming marijuana for me had always been a private endeavor, and many clients who came to me felt the same.

Although I wanted to be a rational voice in the field, I also took the privacy of my patients very seriously because I understood that many cannabis users' reputations and jobs were at stake. Along with serving professionals such as lawyers and therapists, college professors and physicians, I have advised and provided remedies for police officers and a security agent working for the State Department. (He came to me when his wrist pain and subsequent ineffective treatments prevented his use of a high-powered rifle.) They are not about to walk into a dispensary to buy pot. It can also feel exposing to use or associate with cannabis around people we don't know or trust. Public use of cannabis on a large scale is liberating for many, but I think it does little to dispel stereotypes associated with the drug. The first to embrace it are often those whose reputations, jobs, and public standing are not at stake.

The reason I am open about my work is because it's the professional context of medical marijuana that is still referenced so little in our culture. For many patients, it is a drug of necessity. It is a lifeline for escaping more harmful drugs that have no pop-cultural references whatsoever. For these patients, cannabis is very serious. I frame cannabis not as a stand-alone drug but as a plant *in contrast* to the legal pharmaceuticals cluttering up medicine cabinets and polluting our water systems nationwide.[88]

I am also confident in my education and my experience as a teacher. I am standing on the shoulders of all the scientists, researchers, caregivers, and patients who have provided evidence that this plant is not only medicinal but inextricably tied to our cells and our very consciousness. I spoke on panels and allowed myself to be interviewed by media while I was breaking the law because I truly believed I was doing nothing wrong. I followed local ordinances pertaining to home businesses, which in my town allows a "greenhouse or stand for retail sale of agricultural or farm products raised primarily on the same premises and a home business up to 25 visits per week,"[89] and I paid my taxes.

In fact, my illegal business was more conservative and medically focused than the state-regulated dispensaries. Dispensaries provide a valuable resource for patients, but the regulation of them is not perfect. The dispensaries in my state are required to have armed security guards, but they are not required to know or verify their patients' ailments. The retail clerks are not allowed to guide patients medically (as cannabis is not FDA approved), and often customers see a different clerk each time they enter the facility, making the experience disjointed and unpredictable for the ailing patient. Dispensary regulations also require surveillance cameras and force customers to stand in line with strangers to acquire medicine. If you're standing in line at a marijuana dispensary, then why you are there is not private. It is not the dispensary's fault, but these regulations may be in violation of the privacy rule of the 1996 Health Insurance Portability and Accountability Act (HIPPA), which "protects all *individually identifiable health information* held or transmitted by a covered entity or its business associate, in any form or media, whether electronic, paper, or oral."

I have also maintained that a small fraction of my iconoclastic, art school–educated brain *did* want to get caught. I wanted to push the envelope as far as it would go, because the war on marijuana must end. To believe it is a more dangerous drug than prescription opioids is hypocrisy on the part of health professionals, the federal government, and closeted pot smokers alike. To be an illegal pot user and not fight to reform laws is contributing to institutionalized racism. People of color are up to eight times more likely than whites to be persecuted and prosecuted for this plant.[90] This disparity is costly to society, and it is deeply unjust and racist. It is separating children from their parents and sending otherwise law-abiding adults to jail. As a parent, I could not stand for this. I was using the tradition of civil disobedience to protest this injustice.

My relationship to cannabis is also ambiguous. I do fear how people might judge me, and sometimes I wonder if the ethics I apply to it will be lost in a sea of "big marijuana" churning out as much legal weed as possible to fulfill the bottom line. I do not want cannabis to impair the community or my consciousness and psychological development. I do worry that recommending it to patients will stifle their development as adults if they become addicted. But that's why I sit down with patients and provide fact-based, empathic consultation. I pick or recommend remedies that will help, not hinder. I am also pained by the injustice I observe in a medical system that leaves so many people suffering. Few of us in the industry know the science of cannabinoids, know how to grow and process products to treat patients effectively, can teach that to others, and have a healthy relationship with the plant itself. It was this combination of skills that I was ready to bring to law enforcement if, God forbid, it came to my door. I was certainly ready to bring it to a community panel on the subject. My patient Bob and I found ourselves invited to sit on the panel with a local physician, a drug-prevention specialist, a criminal defense lawyer who focused on marijuana, and a local prosecutor.

I chose Bob because he was a retired Wall Street broker in his late fifties. He was demure and polite, new to cannabis, and he was terminally ill. His doctors had given him less than a year to live. Before coming to the panel, he had had a difficult week because he was coming to terms with his fate. It was beginning to sink in that he was going to die.

His wife had brought him to me and was guiding him in using edibles for his chemotherapy symptoms. Several years before, he had lived in New York City, a few blocks from the World Trade Center, when it collapsed in the September 11th terrorist attacks. Although the source of his cancer was difficult to trace, he was diagnosed with a rare form of leukemia that many first responders succumbed to after working on the site. Recent talks about death had also brought up the guilt he had carried his whole life about losing his family in the Holocaust. Cannabis helped decrease his inhibitions and encouraged Bob to access emotions he'd learned to stifle on Wall Street.

Despite being the star of the panel for his heartfelt story, he had been worried stiff that something he might say would get me in trouble. We stood outside the middle school where the event would be held and went over what to say. His head was bald from chemotherapy and his voice was slow and raspy.

"And where should I say I got the marijuana edibles again, Ezra?" he asked me for the third time.

"You say you got them from your 'caregiver,' Bob, which is true. That's where all patients are to *procure* their medical cannabis—from their medical marijuana caregivers. You can say *I* gave you the recipe, which is also true. Really, you're just there to tell your experience as a patient. I don't think people are looking for holes in your story."

"I would just feel terrible if I said something that got you in trouble. I want to make sure I get my story right."

"I really think you're going to do fine, Bob. I don't want you to worry about me." I was reassuring him compassionately, but internally I was defiant. Medical marijuana was legal in the state. We both had medical marijuana licenses to carry cannabis. He was a terminally ill cancer patient and retiree who had survived the 2001 terrorist attacks in New York. I was helping him reduce symptoms of the chemotherapy that made him feel nauseous. I personally grew the cannabis plants I infused into oil and gave to him. Bob felt better. His wife felt more connected and relieved. I arranged his tie, dusted off my suit, and escorted Bob into the school cafeteria.

The panel fostered some positive debate among the experts, and Bob was able to share his story with the world before he passed away. Few treatments were working, and it was a matter of time before he was unable to fight the cancer in his blood any longer. Cannabis for him was helpful as an appetite stimulant and antiemetic, as studies prove.[91] But it was also a way to enjoy the present while he still had the chance. "Enjoying the present" is not medical terminology, but I think most people would argue that a terminally ill patient should have access to a drug that fosters this. The audience was silent as Bob finished his story.

"At any rate . . . I don't know anything about cannabis. I never tried it before I got diagnosed with cancer. I just know that I haven't laughed like this since I was in high school." The audience and the panel laughed, breaking the tension. I put my hand on his back to comfort him. Vulnerability was new to Bob.

We survived the panel, and Bob didn't get me arrested. But he didn't live much longer. He will be missed.

Not long after the panel, media events became more frequent and more patients called on me. Other growers, like Johnny, thought I was crazy for practicing out in the open. I got a call from a local reporter who was doing an article on medical marijuana and wanted to interview me. She also expressed interest in taking pictures for the article. I was confident in my knowledge of the new medical marijuana law, having read the fifty pages of regulations multiple times in search of all the loopholes, but I wanted a few days to think on it before I let her into my basement garden.

Most cannabis growers wouldn't let anyone—let alone a reporter—into their home to see their grow under any circumstance. According to them, I was opening myself up to police raids and home invasion by weed thieves. I told my wife I was being interviewed, but I hadn't revealed that the reporter was going to bring a camera. I would have to figure out how I felt during the interview.

The session was extensive. She sat with me for over two hours. I spewed forth everything I knew and how I came to know it. Clearly, she was interested in what I did for patients, and I could tell she wasn't out to get me busted. She was fascinated to learn about the endocannabinoid system and wanted to hear more about the scientific studies I'd read. When one has an intelligent, sober conversation about cannabis, the SWAT teams breaking down doors, helicopter raids, and federal jail sentences all seem surreal, sad, and anachronistic.

We talked about the ramifications of having photographs of my personal marijuana grow published in the paper. She was all for it. I had trepidation, but my artistic mind was turned on by the idea. What better way to push the envelope, as well as reduce the stigma of cannabis, than to show how innocuous a legal grow—and grower—are? I called my lawyer to double-check the law, and three days later pictures of me and my plants were all over a three-page spread in the paper. After the article, more patients called on me, desperate to find relief where conventional medicine had failed them.

The only activity from police after the article was a call from a local constable who was so miserable on the opioids taken for his back pain that he called me for help. We were each wary of being turned in by the other. We soon realized that we were men of our word, the interaction would be confidential, and his medical needs were greater than the consequences we both feared. I spent most of my sessions with him dispelling stereotypes he had about smoking to relieve pain, as smoking was the only aspect of cannabis he had witnessed in his years of pot busts. The illicit stereotype of pot seemed to leave no room in his brain for exploring other methods of ingestion. He was grateful for my expertise and said he'd stand by me if I ever got in trouble. When I did get in trouble, I was not surprised that I did not see him in the courtroom.

The Helicopter Raid

On the morning of September 22, 2015, the fall weather was beautiful. The sky was a sharp blue, framing maple and oak trees that were changing color in my neighborhood. A light, seventy-five-degree breeze rustled the leaves of the cannabis plants scattered around my half-acre yard. By my calculations, they were about ten days from harvest, their resinous flowers ripening to perfection. By looking at the flowers, I could tell that some strains would need to ripen longer and others were dense and sticky, showing purples, oranges, and reds, like the deciduous trees turning color around them. Although a few of my personal plants were tucked among our tomatoes, scattered at the edge of the woods, or stinking up the occasional flower bed, the majority were on my second-floor deck, out of view of the street. These were the medicinal strains for my patients.

At about 9 a.m., when the sun was just beginning to heat up and the dew was evaporating from their leaves, I stepped out onto the deck with David, my full-time assistant. I was running through a tally of chores for him.

"This one just needs to be flushed with plain water from now on. These two can get full nutrients, these should get half. You can take the dead leaves off those in the back. And can you rotate them all one-eighty? I want the sun hitting every branch."

I turned around and David was stooped over, gently holding a cola, the branch that forms the top flower buds of the plant. He was grinning from ear to ear. "I can't believe how big this one is. Just look at it! It's the biggest bud I've ever seen." He sniffed deeply and exhaled with a satisfied groan. He noticed that I was impatiently holding my clipboard at the other side of the garden. "Oh, sorry. I got distracted," he said.

David was no stoner. After a career running nonprofits for the previous two decades, he had retired and was in the process of getting his medical marijuana card when he found me. He had been using cannabis for years to fight his aches and pains and had seen my flyer at the medical marijuana doctor's office in town. Not wanting to continue to buy weed from his twenty-something children, he sought me out. I gave him my standard consultation and sent him on his way with a couple of strains for pain and sleep, but he kept calling. He had never met anyone who geeked out on cannabis as much as I did—and who was sober while doing so. His calls were persistent and the message was the same: "Ezra, I want to volunteer. I want to help you any way I can. I can tell you're different from the other guys. I just want to offer my help, and I'm going to keep calling you until you let me help you."

I couldn't keep him away. Six months later, as we went over the day's tasks on the deck, he was my right-hand man, working over forty hours a week to help me stay on top of growing, formulating remedies, serving clients, and doing the books.

I looked up from my clipboard. "They're lovely, it's true. That one you're holding is the strain I was telling you about for pain. I have a couple difficult cases I'm excited to try it on. It looks like it could be ready for harvest in a couple days. But let's focus, because I have to deliver to Phyllis today. I want to get this to-do list in order."

This was the peak of my medicinal garden and underground cannabis business. I was nonchalant in putting so many plants outside, but I'd grown outside for years. I never hid my garden or the work I did with patients from the community. Even at their biggest—when their smell was the strongest—no one (without a helicopter) knew my cannabis plants were even there. My neighbor, who lived in the house next door to me, was surprised to read about the raid in the paper. As an attorney, he later wrote a letter of support and encouraged me to use it in my defense.

Dear District Attorney,

I do not know the specifics of Ezra's case, but I can say with absolute certainty that in the nineteen (19) months we have been neighbors I have never observed anything that would suggest that any illegal drug activity was occurring at his residence. In fact, I did not even know that he grew medical marijuana. There has never been any unusual traffic to his home. There have never been vehicles or people coming for short periods of time and leaving. As a criminal defense attorney and former prosecutor I am acutely aware of the activity at a residence that would be suspicious of criminal activity. There simply was no such activity.

Sincerely,
Bill Finn, Esq.

It was no wonder that David and I were oblivious to the fact that in three hours, burly strangers with guns and military fatigues would chop the plants down and cart them away in giant unmarked trucks, never to be seen again.

In the weeks before the raid, law enforcement was the last thing on my mind. I would stand with David and Bruce, my garden manager, on the back deck and fret about whether the crop would be enough to supply client needs through the winter. The deck measured a paltry eight by twenty feet. About thirty full-grown plants filled out the space. The goal was to harvest enough cannabis in the coming weeks to serve my patients into the new year while we prepped the basement garden for the winter crop. Every day I saw new patients for diverse ailments, and every day I would receive calls from patients I'd helped who needed more medicine. Once they'd discovered the healing properties of my cannabis remedies, I didn't want to let them down by running out of product. I also worried about paying David and Bruce, both in their sixties. My stress was no different from that of most legitimate business owners.

I left David to his tasks and set off on my errands. A couple of hours later, I got a text from Bruce alerting me that a helicopter appeared to be hovering over my neighborhood. I had heard rumors that the DEA sent out helicopters to look for outdoor cannabis plants, but I refused to believe them. I assumed they were conspiracy theories and took the rumors with a grain of salt. In one conversation with a colleague who warned me to watch out for helicopters, I waxed poetic about my feeling that what was happening in my yard was bigger than me. I had the space and the client need, so I just gardened. The legislature wrung its hands about the height at which razor wire should be installed around dispensary grow operations, while patients suffered and died. What I did in my yard was a bigger experiment in what an individual's cannabis garden would be like if one didn't subscribe to the irrational laws. I knew the law, I just didn't agree with it and found no evidence in what I was practicing to back up its efficacy. I was genuinely helping people and felt entitled to do so.

And like many iconoclasts, I also didn't fully absorb the possibility that a raid and its aftermath would mean serious consequences for my family. I thought about the families of my students who did not have the resources to fight a similar battle. I believed in the ability of cannabis to heal and help, and I was willing to take that belief to court. Besides, with medical marijuana legal in the state, what rationale would federal agents—or whoever was driving these spying helicopters—have to search a citizen's private yard in a residential neighborhood? Certainly, there was a more efficient use of our tax dollars. FDA-approved opioids were killing people on a daily basis.

I texted Bruce that I was sure it was a training flight originating from the air force base south of town. I wasn't at home, so I didn't hear the cacophony of war machinery rattling windows in adjacent neighborhoods. (Later I was told that neighborhood groups' e-mail threads lit up, trying to get to the bottom of the military-style "attack" they were witnessing.) Twenty minutes later, David called to let me know that the police were at my door. When he called, I was driving to deliver a topical cannabis oil to Phyllis, an eighty-four-year-old client who later told the prosecutor it was the only thing that has worked for her chronic osteoneuropathy. I didn't typically deliver to clients, but as she was homebound, I made the hour-long round-trip to touch base. I always asked if her dose needed to be altered and gave her a big hug. Early on in our relationship, after railing against the pharmaceuticals that made her feel horrible and nearly killed her, she told me she had contemplated ending her life. The pain and lack of mobility were unbearable.

"So do the opioids at least take the edge off the pain?" I asked her.

"They don't even touch it. And they make me feel horrible. I'm like a zombie and can't get out of bed all day long. Your oil is the only thing that works to take the edge off. I put a little bit on my hip every night before I go to bed. I can sleep, and in the morning I can vacuum my apartment. I can walk around. I feel better."

Naturally, hearing that the police had come, I turned around en route to Phyllis and headed home. This was the moment I had subconsciously been waiting for. I parked in the driveway, got out of my boring station wagon, and walked over to the plainclothes officer who was approaching me.

"Hi, I'm Ezra Parzybok, the homeowner." I put out my hand and smiled, looking him in the eye. His hand still holding mine, he stared at me for a full second before responding. I think in that moment I changed the trajectory of my case. Apparently, he had never met a marijuana kingpin as polite and professional as I was. I knew I was thoroughly busted, but I didn't act guilty.

"What do you do for a living?" the officer asked.

"I'm a medical marijuana consultant." I reached into my shirt pocket and handed him a business card.

Within an hour all my cannabis plants, all my jars of oils, tinctures, balms, salves, edibles, dried flowers, and raw leaves for juicing and tea had been confiscated. None of the officers had ever heard of me. Since I had been on local panels and in the paper, many people assumed that my public presence was what tipped them off. But there was no sting operation. It was the helicopter that found me. The DEA funds thousands of similar helicopter searches all over the country and eradicates millions of plants from private homes and yards every year.[92] Many citizens lose their homes and assets for similar crimes. Luckily, I was not arrested or harassed during the raid, but I was told I would receive a court summons in the mail.

In one surreal moment, the officers asked me to come back into the house and explain to them what I was brewing in my workshop. My family occupied a two-family home, and I used the second-floor kitchen and pantry as my apothecary. "We're not asking you to incriminate yourself—we're just curious what all this stuff is. What are you cooking here?" one asked, as I sheepishly entered the kitchen. They all seemed to be over six feet tall and broad shouldered.

I managed to put on my teacher's hat but still felt like a kid showing the judges my lame science fair exhibit. I pointed to a Crock-Pot. "Well, that's a coconut oil paste I am cooking for some cancer patients. You make anal suppositories out of it, which helps reduce the psychoactivity of the THC. These bottles here are actually CBD oil—CBD is a nonpsychoactive cannabinoid used for inflammation, pain, and anxiety." I didn't mention that I bought CBD concentrate legally online and infused it into oils. No use splitting hairs. It was all the same to them. "The other one there is a tincture formula that can be used for micro-dosing—taking in small amounts—to prevent things like migraines, manage chronic pain, or buffer mood swings. That one gets cooked for many hours to break down the THC a bit, which makes it good for insomnia. None of this has been verified by the FDA, by the way, so don't quote me on that."

They all laughed. I was trying to make everyone feel comfortable. They were "guests" in my home, after all. Inside, my heart was breaking, my stomach was tying in knots. Before they packed up, a policeman turned to the detective in charge and asked if he should file a 51A report. Law enforcement is mandated to report drug crimes to the Department of Children and Families (DCF) if children are found living at the location of the crime. I knew that mandatory 51A's filed by social workers, law enforcement, and even their teachers were what resulted in the legal separation of my students from their children when weed was found in their homes. The detective glanced at me where I stood a few feet away, then back to the officer. He nodded briefly and walked away. This is when the reality set in. For the first time since I started growing marijuana seven years earlier, my children were in danger.

Several hours later I was sitting alone in my house, waiting for my wife to come home so I could break the news. As I slumped in a chair, hollow inside, my phone rang. It was Phyllis. "Did you forget about me, Ezra?" she asked. I hadn't forgotten about her. In fact, I had begun to think about many of my patients like Phyllis who depended upon me. I would now have to ask my patients for their help. My moment confronting the justice system had come. If I wanted to keep my family together, I would have to convince the prosecutor of what I believed to be true about medical cannabis. I began collecting letters of support. Here is the letter my seven-year-old son sent to the Department of Children and Families:

Dear DCF,

My dad is respectful & nice. I love my Dad. I don't want to leave my home. They comfort me & secqre [sic] me.

Sincerely,
Marzden Parzybok

The Important Questions

Just a few days after I had given the state police, the National Guard, and local law enforcement an impromptu cannabis class in my home, I was sitting with my family around the kitchen table discussing our unpredictable future. My wife of ten years, our nine-year-old daughter, and our seven-year-old son were eating a healthy breakfast before school, as we always did. But today we were discussing the notion that the DCF might remove our children from the home in which they were both born. Although medical marijuana was legal, and I was a card-carrying patient, distribution of a Schedule I substance in the presence of children constituted "parental neglect."

The night before, I had gotten off the phone with a family lawyer specializing in DCF cases. I was trying to keep the tone of the conversation with my kids as measured and light as possible, but I couldn't shake a comment she had made. If I had been "brown-skinned and living in [a larger city located nearby]," my kids would have been taken away within twenty-four hours. My legal situation was very real.

My kids have always known about the cannabis in our home. They also knew that I made my living as a self-proclaimed cannabis consultant who advised patients on safe and effective use of the drug. My children were as bored with my profession as most children are with their parents' jobs. With my interviews in local media, my lectures on cannabis in the community, and the stream of elderly and sickly clients who came to my home office for consultation, my children found my connection with cannabis to be about as shocking as an accountant's connection with paperwork.

I explained to my kids that the DCF would be coming to the house to interview them. Strangely, they were excited about it. They were articulate, well adjusted, and had nothing to hide. Certainly they would pass the interview with flying colors, they thought.

"So can we do a pretend interview? What are some of the questions?" asked my daughter.

"Yeah, what are the questions? Can I practice my interview? Please!" pleaded my son.

My wife and I exchanged glances. The weight of the situation was growing in our minds like a dark and malignant tumor. I cleared my throat and took on the serious tone of a case worker.

"Okay. . . . Has either of you ever touched the marijuana your dad had in the home?"

My son blurted out proudly: "Oh, I know! Yes, one time my dad let me cut some leaves off his plant in the yard!" He was going to ace this test.

My heart sank, along with my wife's. The raid on my home had already made the front page of the local paper. I pictured the new headline: "Area Man's 7-Yr.-Old Involved in Drug Operation." I knew exactly the moment my son was referring to. The previous summer, I had been harvesting a three-foot-tall cannabis plant from the garden when I let my son cut off a few fan leaves with electric scissors. He was more interested in the scissors than in the plant and eventually moved on to other "weeds" in the garden upon which he could test them.

In that conversation with my kids, it became clear to me that *perception*—not facts, or science, or safety—defined the marijuana debate. We have laws designed to keep children away from dangerous parents, and we have the harmless act of helping a parent in a flower garden. When it came to child safety and medical cannabis, was there no gray area? Thousands of children die every year in America from eating poisonous products in the home or ingesting prescription pills that cause a fatal overdose.[93] My son could have safely eaten every leaf that he cut off that plant. In fact, since cannabis is effective for pain, it's interesting to note that FDA-approved pain medications are the single most frequent cause of pediatric fatalities reported to Poison Control.[94] Yet the worst thing that could happen to a seven-year-old boy eating raw pot leaves is a woozy feeling followed by a long nap—that is, if he could stand the bitter taste long enough to ingest all of them. Whether eaten or smoked, a direct cannabis fatality has never been confirmed.[95] It doesn't shut down organs or cause fatal stomach bleed-outs like opioids or over-the-counter painkillers. It just doesn't work that way in the body.

But *am* I neglecting my children? Are they and my community harmed by the legalization of cannabis? Even though my children attended the school that defined the "school zone" I lived within (and that would affect the severity of my sentencing), what should my punishment be for growing and distributing marijuana? It is infiltrating its way into every community and the medicine cabinets of grandmothers everywhere. Whether we are talking science or perception, illegal or underground, the cannabis industry is literally growing across the nation. We as a culture have concerns. Parents, communities, police officers, prosecutors, and judges who oversee cases like mine are seeking answers. As a parent and cannabis consultant, I take these questions very seriously and have dedicated chapters 3 and 4 to answering them. But in my opinion, there is a more pressing issue in our communities: the tragic suffering of patients. Many citizens who are supportive of marijuana legalization but who are not ailing with acute, chronic, or terminal diseases may not understand the important role cannabis can play in bringing relief to these silent sufferers. Dispensaries without a medicinal approach may leave them suffering. And those with no relationship to cannabis need to understand that although cannabis will be used recreationally, to keep it illegal or restrict its use by the infirm is the real crime. When states do legalize cannabis, addressing the needs of patients should be the primary concern of legislatures, for it was my stories of caring for adults that convinced the prosecutor that medical marijuana was not only real, but necessary.

two

At Their Wits' End

The art of medicine is long, and life is short; opportunity fleeting;
the experiment perilous; judgment flawed.

HIPPOCRATES

Most of my patients in the early days of my practice were adults fifty and older, with serious ailments, who mainly wanted more information on the subject. They had not explored pot in their youth. They spent much of their adult lives managing symptoms and contemplating invasive medical treatments, the results of which were unpredictable. As a parent, I don't feel that the debate about kids and pot is fully settled. But as I hope my patient stories reveal, the risk cannabis poses to youth is worth it, considering what so many people have to endure every day. Doreen, a chronic pain patient, was a case in point. She called me a few weeks after I put a flyer in the local medical marijuana doctor's office.

Doreen's Last Request

"Hi, my name is Doreen and I don't even know how to say this, but I heard about you and I don't have any idea what I'm doing. I think I really need your help."

"Hi, Doreen. Thanks for your call. I assume you're calling about a cannabis consultation?" I replied politely.

"Uh—yes. I don't even know if I'm supposed to say the word or whether that's going to get you in trouble or what, but I've never even tried marijuana. I've been in Alcoholics Anonymous for twenty-five years and I don't want to get high, but I've tried everything else for my pain and I just don't know where else to turn."

Doreen and her friend Jen came to my home office a few days later. Doreen was an elegant woman in her late forties. She had high cheekbones, long blonde hair, and beautifully manicured nails. Her outward appearance was what I would soon learn many chronic pain sufferers look like to the world—very well put together to hide the suffering they live with every day.

"I hope it's okay I brought my friend Jen. I just didn't know if I could trust you or not. You never know."

"I fully understand. Nice to meet you, Jen. The legal gray area makes things very awkward. And most of the caregivers dispensing advice—and marijuana—are doing it out of a parking lot. That's why I'm here. We can talk all we want. I want to make the experience as comfortable for you as possible." I directed them to a couch and chairs in my home office, a sitting area near the front door that was closed off from the rest of the house.

Doreen began to tell her story. At age nineteen, she had been struck by a car, which broke more than sixty bones in her body. She had had so many surgeries that she lost count (she stopped counting after her fifteenth). Although some of the surgeries helped, others caused nerve damage and forced her to use a wider array of opioids to quell the pain. She cried several times during our consultation and eventually had to stand because the pain was so severe. She needed relief but didn't want to reset her sobriety clock by smoking marijuana. She was scared that getting "high" would make her lose control and start drinking again.

"I just don't know what to do. I take about twenty different medications. I have a $500 per month fentanyl patch on my back and it barely works. My sobriety is important to me. I still go to meetings. But I was talking to Jen a couple weeks ago, and I told her that I just don't think I can go on anymore. I told her that I think I'd rather not be here than keep living this way. All I want to do is be able to walk my dog around the block one last time. And then I'm done." She dabbed carefully under her mascara. Jen placed her hand on Doreen's, and they both looked at me sheepishly. Doreen's secret was out.

I took a deep breath, trying to dismiss the idea that I, a self-proclaimed cannabis consultant, was all that stood between Doreen and suicide. I was reminded of all the stories and similar situations I'd had teaching teen moms: abuse, death, suicide, drugs, violence, overdose. You get used to it.

"First, I'm so sorry you have to suffer, Doreen. I can only imagine what you're going through.... You *look* great! So you manage to hide it pretty well," I winked to break the tension a little. "I get that your sobriety is important. We can work with that. I'll also talk about the science of why cannabis can help for pain. Then we can have the legal conversation as well." Her case was daunting, but the challenge was intriguing. This wasn't a stoner seeking to treat her back pain where a yoga class would do. Doreen was at her wit's end. This was my chance to shape her perception of her ailments—and her prospects—with the help of my homegrown "sculptures" I grew in my basement. I was still transitioning in my mind from art teacher to grower to healer.

"Your pain, Doreen, is a perfect symptom for cannabis to combat. Here's a good way to think about it. Say you stub your toe. A pain message gets sent from your toe via nerve receptors to the brain, telling you "ow-ow-ow"! The body's immune system sets off an inflammatory response. Healthy cells go into inflammation mode, and the area swells. Eventually, the nerve cells receiving the pain message naturally release a chemical called anandamide. This is a chemical almost identical to THC, the chemical in the marijuana that gets you high. When the anandamide latches onto the firing cell, the cells get the message to calm down, to *chill out.* The natural cannabinoids in our body are actually designed to regulate cell behavior. Since you have chronic pain, yours keep yelling "ow" over and over again. My hope is that the plant cannabinoids can calm your cells." I gestured to a small cannabis plant I had growing on the window sill.

"So we actually produce a chemical like THC naturally? I didn't know that," said Jen.

"Yes. It's totally crazy, but this is the reason the chemicals in the cannabis plant can latch onto our cells and help us. Although it's fun to speculate about the connection, it's a coincidence of evolutionary biology that this plant makes nearly identical cannabinoids as those we produce in our bodies. And this is why we have a five-thousand-year history of humans using cannabis medicinally," I said.

"That's fascinating. Now I won't feel guilty smoking pot!" laughed Jen. She was warming up to me.

"Easy for you to say." Doreen scowled. "I don't want to get high."

"Absolutely. Your sobriety is important, Doreen. So is your morale. So what's key is to go as slowly as possible and be very conservative. You don't have to smoke it. And you don't have to get 'high' necessarily. I recommend a cannabis oil infusion." I stood up and pulled a jar out of a cabinet containing various strains and remedies. I opened the jar up and set it on the coffee table in front of us. Jen picked it up and smelled it.

"It's what people might typically use for cooking into pot brownies. The coconut oil is cooling to the body, so it's anti-inflammatory as well. You can take such a small dose that on a scale of one to ten, you're maybe at a one or two in terms of being high. It's called microdosing. Over time, the cannabinoids get into your system and help with the pain, but you don't feel it narcotically. It's not physically addictive the way alcohol or opioids are. If you feel at all uncomfortable, just stop. Or take half as much the next time."

"So I just eat the coconut oil? How much do I start with? How long will it take to feel it?"

"Just start with a pea-sized amount. It's less than an eighth of a teaspoon. Wait a few hours to see how you feel. If you feel nothing, then the next day try two peas' worth. Be patient. Only take enough to get results. If you take it and feel it, but it does nothing for your pain, then at least you tried it." I gave a sympathetic smile. "But I'm confident we'll get you some relief." I was beginning to get excited by the challenge of a medical marijuana patient who had exhausted everything allopathic medicine had to offer.

"Okay. This makes sense. So I'm ready to try this. Can I just buy it from you or what?" Doreen held the small jar between her French-manicured fingers.

She was a registered medical marijuana patient. I was, too. (My use of antianxiety medications had secured a recommendation for medical marijuana from a doctor.) We could both legally possess up to ten ounces of cannabis each, which is enough to make about twelve gallons of cannabis oil—about 1,500 jars like the one she held in her hand. But the state wouldn't let us buy or sell it.

"Okay, if you don't have any more medicinal questions, now we can have the legal conversation. Medical marijuana is in a legal gray area. My philosophy is this: you're an adult. You're clearly in pain. You are trying to *avoid* getting high. I believe it is your right to have access to a nontoxic medicine without having to get it off the street or from your doctor. If you want to register me as your caregiver, we can do that. We would both submit separate paperwork to the state. The process takes a few weeks. In some ways, it puts me and maybe both of us at more risk legally. No one really knows, as the law is new. So as they did in California in 1996 when they legalized medical marijuana, we can say that I am just giving this to you for free and you can make a 'donation.' But I only do what my patients are comfortable with. It's up to you."

"Screw it. I don't care anymore. Just tell me how much the 'donation' is. Do you take a check?" Doreen, like every patient I had, grabbed for her checkbook without a second thought.

"You know it's my doctor who told me about you," she said as she wrote the check. "He's the one that's given me all these opioids that I hate. He doesn't know what to do with me, but he knows about you. He wouldn't say your name, but he wrote your name on a piece of paper and then told me he was going to leave his office for a few seconds. And if I wanted to look at the paper, I could. So that's how I had the guts to call you."

I received many clients this way. The doctor is the head of pain management at a Massachusetts hospital. The hospital follows federal law and does not support medical marijuana.

I put the jar in a little gift bag with a patient information sheet I had written up and a receipt for both our records. I took her check (another underground drug dealer no-no that I ignored) and sent them on their way.

Doreen left exhausted from sitting and unsure of the new world she was entering. But she left with hope. That alone took an edge off her pain. In a few days I sent her a text message asking how she was doing. She responded within a few minutes. "Hi Ezra. Well it tastes pretty bad but I take it before bed and I've been sleeping better. One day I took a little too much, but it didn't make me start drinking or anything like I thought it would. I just sort of fell asleep. Pain is still bad but sleeping is a big plus! I will be so happy if this helps me bc there has been no hope for me for years. Thx."

It sounded as if Doreen was easing into the experience appropriately, and she was finding relief. After talking with her, I set out to make another concoction that would perhaps get to her pain faster than the slow-acting coconut oil. She told me that if she could take something before the pain got severe, it would often quell it before it got unbearable. I made an alcohol tincture infused with a mixture of several sativa strains that she could put under her tongue during the day for pain relief. The pain made her exhausted, so sativa varieties might provide a little energy for the day.

"I'll give this tincture a shot. Thanks." Jen wasn't with her for this visit, but I could see her big German shepherd in her back seat. I told her about the dog walk near my house where she could walk it off leash.

I didn't hear from Doreen for several weeks, until I received a thank-you card in the mail:

Ezra,

I just wanted you to know that after close reflection of the past couple of months, my pain level has been significantly reduced. I no longer wear a pain patch, which was very expensive, and I am taking almost a third less pain pills. Even my husband, who was very nervous about [cannabis], sees a big change. My mother thinks it's a miracle because she has been praying to some saint for a few weeks. I think the saint has been helped by me taking your product!

My pain has not gone away but my "very bad, no good days" are far less than what they were before.

—Doreen

Anointed before Dying

Ayurveda, being a sister science to yoga, is a form of medicine that integrates physiological, emotional, and spiritual elements. To approach a patient *spiritually* is to treat a disease as something larger than the sum of his or her ailing parts. Cannabis fits well into the Ayurvedic model because although a drug may have measurable physiological effects, it is difficult to separate our emotional or psychological response to it. Because of its legal status, cannabis is rarely associated with remedies prescribed in Ayurvedic treatments today, but cannabis and Ayurvedic practitioners share a common medium for delivering medicinal herbs: oil. Ayurvedic oils made from almonds, sesame, coconut, and medicinal plants have been used for thousands of years to cleanse, balance, and rejuvenate patients inside and out. The practice of applying medicinal oil to patients—or anointing as Jesus and his disciples did—is called an *abhyanga*. It means to smear or anoint with specific hand movements.[1] According to the *Encyclopedia of Ayurvedic Massage,* it is "designed to deeply penetrate skin, relax the mind-body, break up impurities, and stimulate both arterial and lymphatic circulation, enhancing the delivery of nutrients to starved cells and the removal of stagnant waste. The desired result is a heightened state of awareness that will direct the internal healing system of the body."[2]

Scientific studies are being conducted to demonstrate the measurable health effects of Ayurvedic massages on patients. A recent study concluded that warm oil massage treatments for ischemic stroke victims resulted in improved nervous and cardiovascular system health.[3] Adding cannabinoids, as the ancient Ayurvedic practitioners did, could compound the medicinal benefits. Cannabinoids are created in the plant's fat-soluble or lipid-based resins. These resins dissolve nicely in most oils and in turn penetrate the fatty lipids of our cells. Although our culture has developed a negative connotation to oily and fatty foods, healthy oils are essential to our body. The lipid fats and oils in our body make up cell structure, store energy, and help lubricate all the moving parts in our body.[4]

I frequently advise patients to apply cannabis oil topically based on these modern and ancient principles. I tell my clients that although we take our cars in for an oil change every three thousand miles, rarely do we think to replenish and rejuvenate the oils in the vessel that carries us around—our own body. We don't need scientific evidence to back up the idea of feeling relaxed by a warm oil massage, but in a National Institutes of Health study on Ayurvedic massage it was found that "Subjects showed high statistically and clinically significant reductions in subjective stress experience."[5] Coupled with the right proportion of cannabinoids, a cannabis oil massage could be a transcendent experience for a sufferer of stress, pain, and other ailments. It also helps to note that in Sanskrit, the word for love—*sneha*—means to nurture or to love as well as oily or unctuous. Applying oil to the body is applying love.

Long before I knew of the history of anointing with cannabis oil, I witnessed its effective use on my client David. I was approached by David's wife Wendy, who was a fierce advocate for her husband. She was whip smart, had been a political mover and shaker for many years, and was David's primary caretaker. I was somewhat new to cannabis consulting and, like David and Wendy, had heard about using cannabis for cancer treatment. But I knew only the basics. Some clinical evidence suggested cannabinoids could reverse cancer cell proliferation, and thousands of anecdotal stories online referred to its efficacy in treating or reversing individual cancers. We were not naive enough to think that marijuana was going to magically reverse David's terminal leukemia. But the other drugs David was taking were experimental and not working well, either. He hated popping pills, as they had frustrating side effects. He suffered from insomnia and gastrointestinal issues. Mood swings ensued, distancing himself from those who cared for him. One drug seemed to cause a painful rash all over his body.

I heard that patients who had been successful treating the symptoms of cancer had taken high THC concentrates, but I knew I had to ease David in gradually. At almost eighty years old, he was frail and had been sensitive to medications his whole life. Wendy rolled her eyes when she recounted his pot-smoking years earlier, as one hit could usually knock him out for hours. If one hit was going to make him feel uncomfortable, a concentrated cannabis resin was going to be too strong. I assumed a good solution would be to deliver a lighter dose of cannabis-infused coconut oil sublingually and assess how he felt after several hours.

In my overconfidence, I suggested I deliver the dose in our first session so that they could both see how conservative I was with it. Wendy was driving him home, so he would spend the rest of the day on the couch determining if he felt anything at all. My goal was to get his tolerance up over the next several days and weeks in order to try the more concentrated version of cannabis on him. Like many chemical therapies used to fight cancer, high doses are what often work. Some cancer patients take around 1,000 mg of THC every day for ninety days and attest to its miraculous anticancer and palliative benefits. One thousand milligrams of THC to a sensitive patient would be such an extreme trigger to the ECS that the individual would mostly likely feel debilitating side effects, such as a panic attack, racing heart, lack of balance, and extreme delusional paranoia. It could lead to a temporary crisis of identity, as the user loses control of his thoughts and physical sensations.

I opened a small jar of cannabis-infused coconut oil (identical to the one I gave to Doreen) for them both to inspect. With a butter knife, I scraped off such a small amount of the congealed oil that it was difficult to believe it would have any effect at all. It was about the size of a pinky nail and made the number of "doses" in the jar seem immeasurable. The amount I gave David contained about 2 mg of THC.

Six hours later, I received a call from Wendy that David was in the middle of one of the stronger pot-induced panic attacks he had ever had. He knew he wasn't going to die, but he was not having a good time at all. I felt bad for him and realized there was an even wider spectrum of "conservative" marijuana use than I realized. Many people like David can't handle THC in even small amounts. The episode lasted another six hours, and we determined that it would be a nearly impossible feat to build his tolerance up to a level where he could handle large doses. He had been given a few months to live and wanted to keep trying to deliver cancer-reversing cannabinoids to his system. But he also wanted quality of life. The chemotherapy made him sick enough. No sense adding panic attacks to the equation.

As I discovered through working with many clients after David, in patients' initial uptake of the dose of cannabis, they can feel the euphoria and symptom relief. Within an hour their bodies were often relaxed and comforted by the effect. They, like David, knew intuitively that it was helping morale at the very least. But then the full effect kicked in. Their hearts pounded. Muscles were slack, keeping them paralyzed on the couch. They began to worry that they were having a stroke or dying, and the inevitable paranoia compounded their fears. A tiny bit of cannabis can pack a punch.

I knew that most growers threw away the raw leaves they removed from the plant because they have too little psychoactivity. Since David couldn't tolerate anything else, I suggested that I bring over some raw, leafy cannabis greens, and Wendy could experiment with putting them in a salad or making a smoothie out of them. David was one of my first terminal patients and certainly the most sensitive to cannabis. I liked them both, and they trusted me, but I was not confident that he was going to get much in the way of positive results. We had let go of curing his cancer at this point.

A couple of weeks later, Wendy put me in touch with a hospice nurse named Theresa who had been working with David on the night shift. She explained how she placed a handful of cannabis leaves in a quart of olive oil and cooked it on low heat for several hours. She then strained the oil, and each night she would massage the warm oil into David's body, covering his chest, back, arms and legs. Her technique was probably very similar to what Jesus and other ancient practitioners applied to the infirm. An hour after his massage, his body felt tingly and relaxed. He would drift off to sleep and awake refreshed and happy. Each night the oil was applied, and each morning David felt more joy and was more able to connect with his family during waking hours. The leaves, unlike the stronger THC, seemed to give him energy in the day, but he never felt stoned. The experience was almost spiritual for him. The nurses, Wendy, and his family were grateful for the ease in David's suffering.

This did not cure David. Cancer is complex and tenacious. His leukemia was in an advanced stage and being treated unsuccessfully by the area's top experts. But the experience of the warm cannabis oil on his body was the opposite of what he experienced going in to cancer clinics and doctor appointments. In clinics, he was poked and prodded under bright fluorescent lights. Data-driven doctors looked at his charts more often than they looked him in the eye. The modern treatment for his disease was aggressive, but it was also confusing. Some doctors pointed to their expertise and assessment of the data but contradicted other doctors who were also advising David. The doctors could be arrogant and defensive at times. For David—and for many cancer patients—this experience was devoid of empathy and genuine healing. A cannabis oil massage before bed was nurturing and comforting. It was a soothing, loving touch with a medicated oil. The light dose of cannabinoids was being absorbed into his skin, relaxing his muscles, easing his chemotherapy-induced neuropathic pain, eliminating his rash, and lifting his mood. Just because Jesus and Ayurvedic practitioners found that it eased suffering thousands of years ago doesn't mean that it isn't applicable today. Sickness needs data and the scientific method, but it also needs nurturing and compassion. How might cancer clinics transform the experience of their patients with the medicinal practices of Jesus on their side?

David lived a few months longer than what the doctors predicted, and many of the side effects from drugs were reduced. He passed away surrounded by loving family and caretakers, all of whom witnessed the healing effects of the cannabis oil.

Dale's Skepticism

For some patients, preconceived notions of the drug pose more of an obstacle to health than the dangers of concentrated cannabis. A tragic case I worked with was a seventy-eight-year-old man who had taken a fall when he was shoveling snow. He had hit his head and become paralyzed from the neck down. Sadly, nerve pain left him in agony all over his body, like a vindictive curse. I never met Dale, but his wife Patty came to me as a last resort. He'd been a barber all his life. Now, stuck in a hospital bed in front of the TV twenty-four hours a day, Dale's pain was bad, but his attitude was worse. He had absolutely no faith in cannabis despite the failure of every conventional drug he tried to ease his pain.

"It hurts him when I put his socks on and it hurts when I take his socks off. His skin hurts all over. I've never heard Dale curse like he does when I get him dressed, or God forbid, when we try to bathe him. He's a wreck," explained Patty.

"I'm surprised you're not a wreck, Patty. That has got to be incredibly challenging for both of you," I said.

"Well, it's just what you do. You try to keep going. He was such a nice man before. Now all he does is yell at me every time I touch him. I just don't know what else to do. He most certainly won't smoke it. And I couldn't possibly rub the topical kind on him. It's too painful."

I showed her a vegetable glycerin tincture I had created without heating the THC. "If the THC is never heated then it doesn't get you high, but it can still have anti-inflammatory effects like THC. And it's such a light dose that he probably won't feel anything. But sometimes nerves on the skin respond to light doses." She had asked him to try it, and he went on a rant about druggies and hippies and other unmentionable epithets. So one day she just put a few drops into his feeding bag that hung next to his bed.

"Well," she said, "he found out I was doing it and yelled at me that it was a waste of money. That it didn't do anything and to stop giving it to him. That he didn't believe in quackery."

"Oh, well. That's unfortunate. Maybe if he could take it at higher doses it might help. But obviously you can only do what you can. He's helpless enough as it is. No sense forcing him to try it."

"Yeah, but the funny thing is that the whole week every one of his aides said he was in a better mood. Every one of them said he didn't complain as much when they had to move him."

Dale's case was satisfying from a clinical point of view. It meant that he might be getting relief without a change in his perception.

Some patients were getting pain relief as well as a good giggle session with their loved ones. I met many spouses and caretakers who were exhausted from caring for an ailing relative. They snapped at each other, and tensions ran high even as they sat in consultation. I would watch men who had spent their lives building their business empires weep as they brought their wives in to me for treatment. They couldn't fix their loved-one's pain, and it broke their hearts. One elderly couple came back for a second visit in addressing the husband's pain. The pain had made him miserable to be around, according to his wife.

"They should make *caretaker* one of the ailments addressed by medical cannabis!" she joked, half seriously. Her husband's painful neuropathy was brought on by cancer and the subsequent surgery that removed it. He was now in his eighties, and the doctors saved him but added several years of debilitating pain to his life.

She did most of the talking. "In all honesty, I wanted to try the date balls you gave us to see what he was getting into. I tried pot brownies back in college, you know."

She was a retired bank teller in her late seventies with permed white hair, bright red lipstick, and costume jewelry. The date and almond balls I'd infused with cannabis oil were for her husband, but apparently they both took his "medicine."

"We haven't laughed this much since he was diagnosed two years ago! And plus, they really help me sleep. At any rate, I'm amazed how much healthier our marriage is now."

There were more pain cases. My heart ached for the once peppy soccer mom drowned in morphine, the cabinetmaker relegated to the couch and his disability check, the journalist with searing arthritis in his fingers. The more I got to know my patients, the more I realized that what I was doing was not wrong, it was necessary. I felt like an army medic applying tourniquets on the front lines of a battle against suffering. Laws forbidding tourniquets seemed laughable and out of touch. I knew firsthand that the cannabis I illegally distributed to my patients was reducing the use of harmful drugs. Marijuana's potential to disrupt the opioid epidemic has now been confirmed by a scientific study on medical cannabis patients in California: prescribing opiates, in conjunction with medical cannabis, reduces the amount of opiates needed to treat chronic pain.[6]

The medical field threw everything it had at people like Doreen, David, and Dale, but if doctors couldn't solve their issues they labeled them "problem cases." Their doctors tried treatments, but then they just ran out of ideas. I was not curing anybody. I was just giving people another option.

I wasn't just offering medical marijuana, either. I was spending time with my patients and their families. I was getting to know them. I asked what they did for a living. I asked how they perceived their ailments and asked why they thought it was happening to them in order to get them to think deeply about their healing process. I asked if they had a spiritual or religious life to turn to in the worst moments. I liked unlocking their symptoms and psychological barriers like a puzzle in order to bring them relief with plants I grew at home. These patients had spent tens of thousands of dollars on surgery and expensive treatments. They had visited multiple specialists and traveled hundreds of miles to seek relief. But after all of that, they got relief from me, the high school teacher with an art degree and a basement pot garden.

Cannabinoids

Frequently, patients assume that they need to *smoke* marijuana to access its medical benefits. It does work for some, but smoking is a rapid and powerful delivery system for cannabis. One puff may get you high, but it may not address the neuropathy in your foot, for example, as most of the active ingredients are being delivered to the lungs and brain and not to the source of the pain. I often suggest that a patient start out with a topical cannabis oil for one week, to assess the benefits. In the case of an ailment that affects both limbs (as is often the case with neuropathy), a patient can apply a topical to one foot only. After a week or two of application, the hope is that the cannabinoids will penetrate the tissues at the site of the ailment and bring some relief. Since the patient can compare symptoms between the two feet, he or she can assess if the oil is working. If not, the next step would be to ingest the oil in small amounts (or even to apply it topically to the base of the neck where the nerves enter the brain from the spine). Ingesting delivers cannabinoids into the blood stream via the GI tract. The whole body receives the dose, and as the patient increases the dose, the psychoactive response can be felt more so than a topical application to the foot. The patient can assess the benefits of light psychoactivity as it enters the bloodstream. Sometimes this is the right amount for symptom relief. No stronger application is needed.

Other patients have very serious chronic ailments that do not respond to topical applications or ingestible oils. Although I do wonder whether a nightly anointing with warm oil every day for a month or even a year would change the symptom response, everyone has individual health needs. Some patients report that smoking large amounts of concentrated cannabis resin is the only thing that helps them. Concentrates—like hash—are created by dissolving resin off the plant matter or otherwise separating the plant material from the cannabinoid containing resin. Some processes involve solvents such as alcohol or butane. Others require only CO_2 in the processing. Regardless of how it is processed, the end result can be very potent. Some concentrated resins can contain almost 100 percent tetrahydrocannabinol (THC).

As I am conservative in my approach to cannabis, I have done very little for my patients in terms of concentrated and processed resins containing THC. I worry that the concentrates can increase a user's tolerance of THC, leading to the need for more and more cannabis to reduce symptoms. The processing also begins to mimic what is already happening with the pharmaceutical industry. We are taking a natural plant and extracting only the desired cannabinoids to make a very potent formula. It may be such a potent painkiller that nothing is required of the patient in terms of lifestyle changes. This might be a godsend for some, but others who could benefit from lifestyle changes get stuck in a medicated loop. The body is sustained in its lack of health, the symptoms persist, and the drug masks the symptoms. Then more and more concentrates are consumed to bring about symptom reduction. This can be a life-threatening cycle with opioid use. No concentrated form of cannabis will cause a fatal overdose in an adult (unless many pounds of it are ingested at once), but it does leave the patient struggling with increased tolerance. Many current regulations require dispensaries to allow only card-carrying patients to enter, barring friends and family members from learning the process and helping avoid this cycle of increased use. Therefore, I encourage a patient to bring a friend or caregiver when coming for a consultation. I know they will have someone watching their progress.

Another approach I bring to my patients is to explain how the different cannabinoids work in the body. I find when patients have a better understanding of how the molecules are interacting with their own system, they feel empowered and connected to the healing process. THC is famous for getting the user high. It releases endorphins and causes euphoria, but it can also induce anxiety, make the heart race, and cause panic attacks.[7] I had a client who had no experience with cannabis, but in order to address difficult symptoms of anxiety and insomnia she acquired "medical grade" cannabis resin from a dispensary. The bud tender figured that she needed something strong, as she was clearly suffering, so he offered the strongest concentrate available. She went home and took a small quantity, as he had recommended. The concentration of THC in the resin was about 40 percent, which is low for many concentrates. She took an amount about the size of a pinky fingernail—as David experienced with a less potent oil—which caused days of panic-inducing, psychotic symptoms. She came to me wondering if she had permanently damaged her brain, as the nightmares, tremors, and anxiety hadn't abated days after ingesting the cannabis. Her experience was akin to going to the pharmacy with a bad burn and leaving with gasoline and a match to treat it.

When users experience this paranoia, or the "bad trip" of a strong pot brownie, for example, it is caused by too much THC flooding the system all at once. Even though it is a regulating cannabinoid, the body has its limits. For example, THC is a proven antiemetic.[8] It reduces nausea and vomiting. But at high doses it can induce what is called hyperemesis syndrome.[9] Hyperemesis is uncontrollable retching and nausea and can happen to chronic users who ingest high volumes of THC. Although a study of the syndrome shows that it usually takes an average of fifteen years of use to develop hyperemesis, I have advised novice clients who have experienced it as well. It seems that THC, being a regulator, can regulate itself: it allows the user to consume only so much before tipping the scales and forcing the body to reject it.

For people sensitive to cannabis who are also managing symptoms related to mood, insomnia, anxiety, and intrusive thoughts, the idea of ingesting concentrated amounts of cannabis is a terrifying predicament. It is also a poor medical recommendation. Psychotic episodes may not mean damage to the developed adult brain, but at the very least they are damaging to the morale of patients working hard to regain balance and sanity in their lives. Many users who have a high tolerance to THC need all they can get to reduce their symptoms. But most new users either need a more moderate balance, or they should explore other cannabinoids that are mild in comparison.

Cannabidiol (CBD) is the second most prominent cannabinoid present in the plant and has been shown to offset the strong effects of THC.[10] This means that strains higher in CBD will tend to have a decreased psychoactive effect. The research on CBD is recent, but it is very promising. CBD is a muscle relaxant, it has analgesic properties,[11] and it has been shown to reduce anxiety in human and animal test subjects.[12] The CBD content of the concentrate my client took with her 40 percent THC was still 80 percent, much higher than the THC, but even at that level of concentration, both could bring debilitating side effects to a new or experienced user. A typical cannabis flower may have only 20–30 percent THC when smoked. CBD, although an anxiolytic, has increased anxiety in some of my clients at doses of less than 10 mg. These are referred to as the "paradoxical effects" of some medications.[13]

There is not a sufficient comparison to this level of concentration in other alterants such as alcohol or coffee. Taking a small sip of a triple espresso or 190-proof vodka can startle the palate, but it will not get you wired or drunk for days on end. A good comparison to the effect concentrated cannabinoids can have on the system is chili peppers. If you are looking to add a little spice to your burrito and you've never tried hot sauce before, imagine a waiter offering a bite of a habanero pepper. A small bite of a habanero pepper could induce a prolonged chemical burn in the mouth. This amount might be sufficient for making a quart or two of medium to hot salsa. Thus, what makes cannabinoids medical does not mean that they are *more* medical in stronger amounts. I would have suggested that my anxiety client start with a cannabinoid product high in CBD with only trace amounts of THC and ease into it slowly. When we're talking about addressing subtle ailments of the mind, the user has to be brought along slowly, so that the effects of the drug can work *with* the mind to control symptoms.

Anxiety, for example, is tough to pin down as an ailment, but its pathology is clear in our language. We get *nervous,* we have raw *nerves,* we are having a *nervous* breakdown. Even *butterflies in the stomach* or a *gut reaction* point to the trillions of nerves in our gut responding to the worry we feel about a situation. In order for us to calm our nerves, our cells release cannabinoids that are designed to bring the cells back into balance. Enzymes then automatically break down the cannabinoids. CBD, unlike THC, is so subtle that it doesn't latch onto receptor sites in the cells the way THC does. But it does regulate the enzymes.[14] If anxiety is severe, the nerves are on high alert. Our natural endocannabinoids are released but may not have enough oomph to regulate the nervous system. The enzymes are released anyway to dissolve away the cannabinoids, leaving the anxiety in place. CBD can slow the enzymes from breaking down endocannabinoids. My analogy for explaining how THC affects ailments differently than CBD is that THC is like calling the fire department, sirens wailing and boots clomping. It may trigger cell response and be felt rapidly, but like a fire fighter smashing windows and hosing the furniture down, THC may come with stronger side effects. CBD, a subtler change agent, is generally not felt at lower doses, so it is more akin to a social worker or therapist, toning and training the system to get it back on track by itself.

In the decades-old underground pot community in America, CBD was not only unknown, but useless. Its subtle effects were dominated by the much stronger THC. All cannabis breeding was done to increase THC. It was even feared that aggressive breeding would eliminate important cannabinoids, but as CBD has become a sought-after molecule in the medical marijuana community, high-CBD varieties are now being created. Luckily, it is produced in hemp plants as well. The federal government restricts the growing of hemp in the United States, presumably because of the perception that a pot leaf is a pot leaf no matter its cannabinoid content. But it is not illegal to import hemp products to the United States. I buy my CBD in concentrated oil form from a company that grows it in Holland. Incidentally, the DEA has changed its language on CBD in order to crack down on its sale. In late 2016, it made CBD concentrate a Schedule I substance. Unfortunately for them, CBD is still legal because the DEA does not make or change laws. Their classification of CBD will be challenged in court. The DEA challenged the hemp industry under similar circumstances early in this century. As with that court battle, the DEA will most likely lose this one.

Since we don't have specific receptors in our brain for CBD, it is generally thought that CBD is not psychoactive. I have found the CBD I use to be nonpsychoactive in small amounts, but psychoactivity is also a subjective experience. Some who use CBD clearly describe their experience as being "stoned." One way to think of it is that THC gets you "high" whereas CBD gets you "low." Although it has been shown to regulate depression as well,[15] I have found that very high doses of CBD can cause a melancholy or depressed sensation.

Others find it has only a physical effect but doesn't alter the mind or one's cognition. Ideally, when taking CBD, symptoms can feel mitigated, but no strong or "altered" effect is experienced. As with THC-dominant strains of cannabis, I have noticed that CBD has different effects if it is derived from different sources. I have interacted with patients and tried CBD myself that is derived from marijuana strains created in the United States. The sensation is not the "high" of THC, but it is clearly "felt." I am very sensitive to THC myself, and small amounts can cause me to experience anxiety. I have inhaled pure CBD that did not feel like a THC high at all but still made me anxious, as it flooded my nervous system powerfully. A smaller dose, taken orally as opposed to smoked, might decrease anxiety, where an inhaled form might increase it. Thus, it is important to know the source and effect of the product.

The CBD I use with patients has a purity that reflects a reduced high, but I did have an interesting experience with a CBD "overdose." As I was filling a small bottle with CBD concentrate infused in grain alcohol, I spilled the bottle on the counter. My first thought was that I didn't want to waste the CBD: it is very expensive, as it requires many plants to produce a small amount. I had also not taken a large dose before and knew that the alcohol was probably killing any germs it was coming in contact with. I promptly sucked it all up off the counter. The dose was approximately 125 mg of CBD, roughly five to ten times the recommended dose for symptoms of pain or anxiety. Within two hours, the full force of the CBD entered my bloodstream. The first thing I noticed was a confirmation of what I tell patients. Where the cannabinoid enters the body is where it will be felt most strongly. Since it was an alcohol-based tincture, it was absorbed by capillaries in my mouth and throat before it entered my GI tract. My head, neck, and shoulders were heavily sedated. Similar to the effects of taking Benadryl, my whole upper torso felt as though it had been wrapped in a warm, heavy blanket. My mind was so sedated by the CBD that I felt a bit foggy-brained and melancholy. The next several mornings, my usual high-cortisol anxiety was nonexistent. My limbs were rubbery and heavy, and as each day progressed I could feel the sensation spread from my head and upper torso down to my lower torso and eventually to my extremities. Although the heavy dose made me melancholy, verging on depressed, for several days, I also noticed my cravings for alcohol, THC, and sugar to be absent. Some of this craving reduction has been backed up in trials on CBD for drug addiction, including with nicotine, psychostimulants, and opioids.[16] Although the studies on reducing opioid cravings were effective, they have been tried only on mice. The nicotine study was performed on humans and showed a 40 percent reduction in the number of cigarettes smoked. Thus, CBD seems to have an effect on the body that reduces cravings and addictive tendencies. I'm not sure what the DEA is thinking, but a drug that has clinically verifiable results for reducing addiction is a drug that should be legalized, not placed in Schedule I, in my opinion.

As long as a patient has guidance on how to use CBD and does so conservatively, it is a good entry point in terms of medical marijuana. As I will discuss in the next chapter, CBD can also be an effective topical application for muscle convulsions.

Dozens of other cannabinoids exist. A new trend is the use of cannabinol, or CBN. When THC degrades, the molecule becomes CBN, which has demonstrated anti-inflammatory[17] and anticonvulsant[18] effects as well as an ability to fight the hard-to-kill MRSA virus.[19] Although CBN alone showed little effect, combined with THC its sedative effects were demonstrated in human volunteers.[20] Many other studies are being conducted on the action of other cannabinoids such as CBG, CBC, and THCV. In the coming years, research will map out the many medicinal applications of these diverse cannabis-based compounds.

There are also flavors and smells in cannabis called flavonoids and terpenes. Each has a different effect, and according to extensive study on the subject they too can "offer complementary pharmacological activities that may strengthen and broaden clinical applications and improve the therapeutic index of cannabis extracts containing THC, or other base phytocannabinoids."[21] Limonene, for example, the terpene associated with the citrus aroma and is a common terpene in cannabis, has been shown to positively affect depressive symptoms.[22] Many growers I know obsess over growing techniques designed to heighten the terpenes in the plant for their medicinal benefits. As aromas enter the brain directly, they do have potential for fast-acting relief as they easily cross the blood-brain barrier.[23] Their use in medical marijuana is promising, but patients should not assume that smoking a strain called "Lemon Haze" is going to cure their depression. If you want to test the antidepressant effects of limonene, you might start off by carrying a lemon around and sniffing it a few times a day. It's actually quite uplifting, produces no psychoactive effects, and is legal everywhere lemons are sold.

Terpenes are also affected by the curing, storage, and growing environment. As with a fine wine, if these variables are altered, the terpene profile is altered, changing the potential therapeutic effect. In the years to come, all the molecules in cannabis will be studied more in depth and enhanced to create symptom-specific products. THC will be an important aspect of cannabinoid remedies, but with its deregulation, perhaps advocates on both sides of the marijuana debate can seek to reduce THC dominance in favor of a wider spectrum of beneficial cannabinoids and terpenes. With this approach, the stigma surrounding cannabis may decrease, patients will have more nonpsychoactive options, and doctors may open up to its vast medical potential.

The Cancer Conundrum

Lee Young was open to cannabis when he painstakingly hobbled into my consultation office for medical marijuana advice, but his heart was heavy. He had been given just a few months to live. His body was atrophied, his movements slow and methodical from constant exhaustion. But his voice still had a positive lilt, making him seem younger than his sixty-five years. He told me he felt at peace mentally, but he was not naive about his prognosis. In fact, he'd been fighting stage 4 prostate cancer for nearly eight years, living years longer than the doctors predicted. He told me about his ongoing stomach issues and lack of appetite. Because his prostate cancer had moved into his pelvis and spine and now his lungs, he also had chest pain. Breathing had become difficult. The last thing he wanted to do was smoke pot.

He had tried all the conventional treatments over the years and had settled into the soft-eyed soulfulness of knowing his time could be up any day. After cancer was finally discovered in his lungs, his doctor was not mincing words. "It's just a matter of months," he had told Lee several months earlier. At that meeting, his physician recommended he pursue cannabis for symptom relief. Lee didn't know why his doctor recommended it. "Maybe he just thought that since I didn't have much time, the euphoric side effect would help. But my doctor didn't know much about it, didn't know where I'd get it, and couldn't recommend how to use it."

During the Vietnam War, Lee had spent two years living in proximity to an Agent Orange storage facility. It was there that he first discovered cannabis. He frowned upon the pot his fellow soldiers smoked, until he tried it one day to see what the fuss was about. He understood the appeal right away. Although he enjoyed it off and on for years after the military, he hadn't smoked marijuana for about fifteen years when he drove for over an hour to get to me. "I didn't want to buy it off the street. I knew I could get it through friends, but I wanted medical marijuana from a reliable source."

I empathized with Lee and his story, but I didn't mince my words, either. "I'm going to start you with a cannabis-infused oil you can ingest that might ease your pain and help you sleep. Some people say it helps their digestion. But it's not a magic bullet. It's not a miracle cure." I told him that there was some scholarly evidence that cannabis had slowed the growth of cancerous cells in a laboratory as well. There was evidence that it could slow some tumor growth[24] in mice and prevent human cancer cell proliferation[25] in the lungs and some brain tumors[26] of patients with glioblastoma, but I was focusing on symptom reduction.

Many doctors are skeptical that pot can do anything to help cancer symptoms, let alone slow cancer. But my opinion is, if you have mere months to live and are in pain, and there's a nontoxic drug that has been shown to provide moderate cancer cell destruction, as well as bona fide symptom relief of symptoms—from nausea to insomnia—then why would any cancer patient (let alone doctor) turn that drug down?

Doctors have eloquent responses to this question. In my attempt to gather unbiased information, I came across a well-researched blog post by a cancer doctor and blogger.[27] But despite the oncologist's eloquent and objective approach to the data on cannabis research, I did not have much trouble finding the typical holes in his argument. As any researcher would, he was responding skeptically to the numerous sites on the Internet that "prove cannabis cures cancer," and he offered the real facts on cannabis studies: "So while there does appear to be anti-tumor effect against the glioma cell lines tested, it was, at best, modest. Certainly, it wasn't the sort that would knock my socks off as a cancer researcher."

His article is titled, "Cannabis Does *Not* Cure Cancer," but naturally, as someone with empathy and hope for my clients' cancer survival, I was amazed how tone-deaf he came across, despite being someone who specializes in treating cancer patients. Certainly, he's watched families grieve, watched once-strong individuals wither away, and seen women's identities permanently altered by their breast cancer (his specialty). Many patients are desperate, and his statement "There does appear to be anti-tumor effect" would clearly spark hope and curiosity in his patients and their loved ones.

The fact that a single plant—which has been illegal for three generations in this country—might actually have positive health benefits for cancer deserves a moment of pause. This isn't a dietary supplement purporting to offer general health benefits. This is an illicit drug for which clinical evidence shows that it helps fight a disease that affects one in three adults.[28]

For the millions of Americans who have smoked marijuana in fear of persecution, give them a moment of satisfaction that it is now up for debate that it *cures cancer*. But it also compounds the cannabis conundrum. Perceptually, the leap from street drug to cancer drug is too large for many. But there are thousands of anecdotal cases on medical marijuana and cancer patient forums of patients slowing, reversing, or eradicating their cancer entirely with the help of high doses of cannabis.

The process is not simple. Patients can smoke a joint before their chemotherapy session in order to mitigate nausea. But patients attempting to fight back their cancer are taking cannabis as an equivalent to chemotherapy. The "standard" dose of one gram of concentrated THC per day is a powerful amount intolerable to most adults. A special extraction process removes the resin from the plant, turning it into a thick tarlike oil that is ingested or put into anal or vaginal suppositories. The patient eases into higher and higher doses of cannabis, but the idea is that eventually the body can adjust over time. Billions of THC molecules enter the patient's system, with the intended result of essentially turning off as many cancer cells as possible. What has been demonstrated in laboratories is that THC helps induce apoptosis, or programmed cell death.[29] This is a natural behavior that happens to millions of cells in the body every day. When they are no longer needed, something triggers their "death," and they are removed as waste. Due to carcinogens from tobacco or environmental toxins stopping apoptosis, for example, these zombie-like cells can multiply uncontrollably and become tumors or disrupt normal processes in tissues, the blood, and bones. The idea behind cannabinoids and cancer cells is that cannabinoids are *regulating* cell behavior toward homeostasis. If certain cannabinoids encounter a cell that has been proliferating uncontrollably into a tumor, it triggers apoptosis. Tobacco smoke has the opposite effect.[30] That's why tobacco kills about seven million people worldwide every year,[31] whereas researchers have not been able to demonstrate a cannabis and lung cancer link.[32] If your doctor or your school drug counselor tells you that smoking pot is as dangerous as smoking tobacco, they are off base by a factor of many millions. The science is fascinating. But it is also contradictory. The study mentioned earlier, "Cannabis and Tobacco Smoke Are Not Equally Carcinogenic," published in the *Harm Reduction Journal,* finds that "compounds found in cannabis have been shown to kill numerous cancer types including: lung cancer, breast and prostate, leukemia and lymphoma, glioma, skin cancer, and pheochromocytoma. The effects of cannabinoids are complex and sometimes contradicting, often exhibiting biphasic responses. For example, in contrast to the tumor killing properties mentioned above, low doses of THC may stimulate the growth of lung cancer cells in vitro."

Regardless, millions of cancer patients have tried it. Some have been helped and others have not. There are now cancer clinics using conventional as well as high-dose cannabinoid therapy to successfully treat cancer, but it is still controversial. So far, no controlled trials have shown concentrated cannabis oil to be effective in reversing cancer. Taking my model of comparative medicine into account, all cancer treatment must be scrutinized for its efficacy. Not all conventional methods are effective, either. For example, one study of three thousand breast cancer patients found that those receiving radiation in addition to surgery did no better than patients who received surgery alone.[33] As I tell my patients, in order to develop effective treatment for the individual, a patient and his or her doctor must lay out all the forms of treatment, weigh risks objectively, and make an informed decision. The same study says, "The FDA has approved more than 80 anticancer drugs, 40 of which are chemotherapeutic agents. [They] are also neo-carcinogenic which can lead to the development of new cancers that did not exist prior to the administration of chemotherapy." So again, I agree that we should take a conservative approach to whether or not cannabis *cures* cancer, but many cancer drugs are *causing* new cancers. If it is effective for even a single patient, shouldn't cannabis be on the table as a possible treatment when other treatments may also exacerbate cancer? Many of my cancer patients come to me for help treating their lingering chemotherapy and radiation side effects such as neuropathy, gut issues, or insomnia.

There are multitudes of different cannabis trials that could be conducted to address its outcome on cancer in all its stages. Cannabinoid therapy at the onset of treatment, in conjunction with other chemical therapies, different methods of ingestion, or at different concentration or cannabinoid ratios could be tested. The comprehensive study "Cannabinoids as Therapeutic Agents in Cancer: Current Status and Future Implications," which compiled data on the effect of cannabis on breast cancer, prostate cancer, lung cancer, skin cancer, pancreatic cancer, bone cancer, glioma tumors, oral cancer, head and neck cancer, and its many other effects, concludes with this statement:

"Thus, [the] combination of cannabinoids with other chemotherapeutic drugs might provide a potent clinical outcome, reduce toxicity, increase specificity and overcome drug resistance complications."[34]

The data needed to address cancer are more complex than just chemical agents. For example, a study has found that there is also an increase in effectiveness if a patient believes in his or her treatment.[35] Since it has been confirmed that cancer treatment can cause depression, and psychological stress may alter immune function,[36] we need to look at the euphoric properties of cannabis as a viable way of treating a patient's depression during cancer treatment. I know that the medical field and law enforcement are stuck between this clinical evidence and the DEA's stance on cannabis. But doctors have taken a vow to "do no harm." Police are mandated with protecting and serving the community. I implore them to have empathy and the courage to read the evidence and then speak out. Cancer patients and their doctors are the citizens who can change the stance of the DEA.

A couple of weeks after I was raided by the police, my cannabinoid-laden plants ripped from the ground, I bumped into the director of the local marijuana dispensary, which had been open for a few days. Despite rumors that the dispensary had tipped off the police to "squash the competition," he graciously offered to buy me dinner. The dispensary was in no way involved with the raid. During our conversation, he mentioned how much further along Israel was in using cannabis for treatment of cancer in its hospitals. He was Israeli himself and had spent time researching the medical marijuana system there and interacting with Dr. Mechoulam, the Israeli scientist whose success in synthesizing THC first led to the discovery of the endocannabinoid system.

"In Israel, I was told they did a trial in the hospital to determine its effectiveness in treating symptoms of pediatric cancers. They gave five hundred children doses of cannabis oil via an IV, and five hundred children got a placebo. After a few weeks, they had to stop the trial," he said.

"What? Why is that?"

"The children who got the marijuana were doing so much better that they felt it was immoral to go on with the trial."

In my opinion, the scientific data detailing the potential effectiveness of cannabis in reducing the symptoms of cancer treatment, as well as its measured (albeit modest) ability to address the mechanisms of the underlying cancer, make it a viable medication that should always be considered, especially for children. Many cancer patients came to me with prognoses similar to Lee's and little desire to get high. Again, it seemed morally wrong to not help them. I grew cannabis organically. I knew the science. I cared about my patients and spent more time with them than their doctors did, because I could. Doctors I knew sometimes saw dozens of patients a day. I saw one or two at the most.

I walked Lee through using the oil. I told him he could cook with it in low doses, and if he traveled with it, he should just put it with his other medications.

"No one will find it if you don't hide it. It's oil, so they'd have to analyze it to determine whether it had THC in it. It's not a high risk to carry it around. Besides, you're a terminal cancer patient with a medical marijuana card. Law enforcement needs to get over it." He paid me for my time and made the $50 "donation" for the jar of oil. I guided him slowly out to his car, vaguely wondering why I felt I had the authority to help a terminal cancer patient.

Lee and I interacted a few more times, as I advised him in his oil dosage and administration methods. He was sensitive to it and would not be able to acclimate to a highly concentrated dose of THC anytime soon. He mentioned again that he had no intention of smoking, but I had done more research and had some intuition about what might help him. I laid out my hypothesis one afternoon on the phone.

"I have been thinking, Lee. Cannabis relieves pain. This is proven.[37] It also dilates blood vessels,[38] so that could be good for your asthma symptoms. Doctors will tell you there are more carcinogens in combusted cannabis than in cigarette smoke, which is true, but as noted earlier, laboratories have not been able to show these carcinogens making human cells cancerous. One puff a day is unlikely to exacerbate your cancer since it has also shown moderate success in combatting some cancerous tumors. If we could get a light dose of cannabinoids right to your lungs, maybe we could just help you breathe better." I wasn't a pothead telling him that smoking would cure his cancer. I was forming a hypothesis for a single patient.

Maybe the utter lack of medical knowledge I gathered in art school made me think outside the box in treating Lee. The nice thing about working with terminal patients is you don't have much to lose when you try something risky. I told Lee the story of the guy who helped invent chemotherapy. He gave increasingly high doses of a derivative of mustard gas to pediatric leukemia patients until it either killed them or kept them alive. Most of his colleagues thought he was evil and immoral to do it, but the upshot was that it worked.

Lee had few options, so he thought he'd give my hypothesis a try. On a visit, I told Lee to find a calm, quiet setting and remove the pot-smoking stereotypes from his mind. Take a single puff, inhaling and exhaling a normal breath.

"If you hold it in, you'll just cough and inflame your lungs, so don't do that. After you inhale, wait ten or twenty minutes and see how you feel. Repeat again the next day."

He'd actually purchased an expensive vaporizer that I taught him to use, but he hated it. I tend to be a marijuana traditionalist. Smoking pot the old-fashioned way has just not proven to be a health issue, unless you're Johnny, smoking copious amounts every day. Even in cases like Johnny's, it's linked to an increase in chest colds, not lung cancer.[39] So I made him a long wooden pipe with a tiny smoking bowl at the end and selected a strain I grew called Pennywise for its purported cannabidiol (CBD) content. CBD has also killed cancer cells in laboratory experiments.[40] I didn't bore him with the details. I could tell he felt defeated about trying to smoke at all.

"By all means, if you hate it, or if it makes you feel uncomfortable or makes you cough, then stop," I told him. I was kneeling on one knee in my driveway, explaining all of this to him through the open door of his car so he didn't have to get out. I felt confident much the same way children feel confident in their mud pie making, guileless as they present it to Dad. I presented my hypothesis, dripping with sticks and leaves, but full of heart. Thank God his pulmonologist was not within earshot.

A few weeks later, I called Lee up to see how things were going (and also to see if he was still alive). He wasn't in love with the ingestible oil, he said, but he liked to have it applied topically to his chest and spine. If nothing else, the loving touch seemed to help his pain. "That's great," I said. He was in good spirits because his body aches had subsided and his lung pain had decreased significantly. He had smoked a puff or two of Pennywise a day, with no more than three puffs (presumably on a Friday night) at any one time.

He said it didn't get him high. It made him sleepy, but mostly he noticed an openness in his chest. After months of suffering, he could now take a deep, pain-free breath.

Over the next year I successfully used Pennywise to treat a patient's asthma symptoms (also by smoking in light doses with a handmade pipe). Another clinically diagnosed sufferer of severe anxiety inhaled it three times a day with a vaporizer, which allowed her to reduce several psychoactive drugs that caused debilitating side effects. It was one of the more unusual strains I ever grew. Visually it looked like a sativa strain, but its effects were more calming and sedative, similar to an indica strain. Some people also tried the strain and said it didn't get them "high" at all. My wife tried it as well and disliked it, as it put her to sleep too rapidly. I found it sedated my body but kept my mind awake. I marveled that this one plant had such varying results, and I assumed the CBD was playing an important role. I had never used a CBD-rich strain before, so I sent a sample of Pennywise to be analyzed at a laboratory. The flower sample had a 27 percent THC content, a significant amount for any strain, especially one that purportedly had no altering effect on some users. I also discovered something surprising. The strain had a negligible amount of CBD—less than 1 percent. Despite patients reporting its CBD characteristics repeatedly, the cannabinoid analysis did not tell the whole story. Could a strain with a *lineage* of higher CBD content still have CBD-like character-istics even though it had a small amount of the cannabinoid? (The specific variety I grew came from seed, and although other Pennywise seeds can be found, they are not genetically identical to mine.) Since there is speculation that a third cannabinoid receptor may be present in the endocannabinoid system,[41] I wonder if its cannabinoid profile was triggering receptors we haven't mapped out yet. We will never know, as every last vestige of it was eradicated by law enforcement during the raid on my home.

I understand that the scientific method requires rigorous testing, and most research-minded readers will know that one or two success stories do not an FDA-approved drug make. But there is something in bona fide research called an N=1 trial. This is when you perform a trial or test a drug or hypothesis on one person. If it works, then it provides enough evidence to be tried on a larger scale. One of the most famous examples of its success is the N=1 experiment performed by internist Barry Marshall, who speculated that ulcers were caused by bacteria and not stress, as most people thought at the time. Unable to secure funding for his hypothesis, he famously gave himself a bacteria-induced ulcer and successfully treated it. Defying the medical field's skepticism, he proved right, and his N=1 trial eventually led to a Nobel Prize for himself and his colleagues.[42]

As I've mentioned, cannabis is challenging to test because it is a plant subject to different growing conditions and different molecular profiles. The FDA may wring its hands about it for decades. But cancer patients have no time for this. About six months after Lee came to me, he visited his doctor, who reported that the cancer in his lungs was completely gone. Lee speculated that using a light dose of cannabis daily at his lung cancer's early onset was enough to reverse its course. I was ecstatic and curious over the phone. "What did your doctor think? Was he amazed? Was he so happy to deliver the news?" I asked.

"He just . . . gave me the news. He seemed happy, but that was it. He just told me it was gone. I didn't mention that the only thing I had been doing differently was smoking your cannabis once a day," he chuckled. "Well, there's obviously no way to prove it was the smoking, but I'm so happy for you!" I said.

Over a year later, when I visited him for research on this book, we marveled at the irony of my smoking hypothesis. I mentioned that New York State had just legalized medical marijuana. "Though the law prevents any smokable cannabis products from being sold," I said. Lee lived over a year past his last prognosis. He had become so comfortable with using various cannabis remedies effectively that I eventually brought a small cannabis plant to put in his bedroom. Nestled among his other house plants, it looked innocuous. But Lee shared a special bond with it. "I know that cannabis has contributed to giving me more than a year of prolonged life. I am very grateful for that," he told me. When they wheeled his body from his home, the plant remained, basking quietly on the window sill.

Cancer is a pervasive and tragic disease. It will likely be diagnosed in half of adults in their lifetime.[43] Billions of dollars are spent searching for a cure, but the disease is complex and insidious. I am humbled to be sought out by cancer patients for my expertise on cannabis, but I do not profess any miracle cure. As with any dangerous disease, all options, from aggressive conventional treatments to touchy-feely remedies, should be on the table. The best treatments are the ones that work. The layman's explanation of what cannabis does in the body helps elucidate, from a metaphorical perspective, how cancer is both a ruthless and a poetic disease. Cancer is essentially healthy cells in the body that get stuck in a feedback loop of proliferating uncontrollably. Cancer reminds us of an invasive virus multiplying out of control. We talk about wanting to kill the cancer. But it is us—our cells—that are stuck in the cycle. If the cells in our body contribute to the consciousness that makes up who we are as people, then researchers might eventually devise experiments to determine how consciousness might be playing a role in some forms of cancer and its treatment.

I worked with a stage 4 breast cancer patient who had gone through chemotherapy, and who had several surgeries. She also used high doses of raw cannabis suppositories that she said kept her cancer cell count in check. She shared her opinions on the subject readily.

"Every cancer patient I know who is using the raw plant infused in oil as a suppository is feeling better during their cancer treatment. A lot of us do it. We just don't share it with our doctor because they don't understand. I've even gone out to New Mexico to do an ayahuasca ceremony three times. Every time I go, my cancer cell count goes down. My doctor doesn't believe there's a connection. But who cares? I feel better and the cancer count is down!"

I cringe at the idea that someone would use cannabis and forgo conventional treatment. This is a narrow way of thinking, akin to the conventional medical model that does not take into account the emotional well-being of the client or how connected he or she feels to his or her health provider and treatment. If I or a loved one had cancer, of course I would seek out all options. And I would read the results of every scholarly study connected with that treatment before pursuing it. Ignorance can have tragic results. But I believe people diagnosed with cancer should have a wide selection of properly formulated cannabis remedies available to them while they seek conventional treatment.

three

What about the Children?

*It is not enough to say something is legal and that's enough.
What matters is if it is legal and moral . . . if it is legal and responsible.*
EDWARD SNOWDEN | interview in *Pod Save the People,* May 12, 2017

I have witnessed parents detail their children's experience with conventional drugs in my cannabis consultation practice. They teared up as they tallied the harmful side effects wrought upon their loved ones: suicidal thoughts from antidepressants, permanent gut issues caused by the overuse of antibiotics, prolonged brain chemistry imbalances from mood-altering drugs. Others recounted insomnia, night terrors, hospitalizations from drug interactions, or heroin-like withdrawal symptoms from stopping the prescription drugs. These are the tragedies on top of the symptoms and diseases from which their children already suffer.

The Parents' Dilemma

I will address the most common debate concerning cannabis and children: whether smoking pot is bad for kids. It is a debate that elucidates the extreme myopia with which we approach cannabis and youth. We tend to believe cannabis is only about smoking, despite the fact that cannabis is a plant that can take many forms. For a patient, young or old, it can be concocted into countless remedies that bring symptomatic relief without inhalation or making someone high. When it comes to the choice of whether to explore medical marijuana for a symptom or disease, my approach is simple: take the readily available, doctor-prescribed medication for a specific ailment and compare it side by side with the appropriately formulated cannabis remedy. Make an informed decision with your health care provider based on the facts, not perception.

A doctor might respond to my approach by mentioning the lack of studies done on cannabis. He or she might decide there are too many unknowns, and instead take the conservative route—prescribe painkillers to a teenager injured while playing sports, for example. The young athlete will exit the hospital with crutches and a bottle containing enough synthetic opioids to kill a horse. Opioids cause fatal overdoses. They're also worth a lot of money if the teenager doesn't use them all but knows someone who will. Three out of four people who abuse prescription opioids get them from a friend or family member.[1] These are the knowns. We may not know what will happen to that teen if he or she smokes weed to relieve pain over the next few weeks. But it can't kill them. Prescription drugs can. According to the Centers for Disease Control, between 1999 and 2015 prescription opioid overdoses accounted for 183,000 deaths.[2] And every day, more than a thousand people are treated in emergency rooms across the country for using opioids improperly.[3]

Yes, cannabis has addictive properties—but not as much as opioids or even alcohol. It has been estimated that 25 percent of patients who receive opioids struggle with addiction.[4] Alcohol, ubiquitous in nearly every home, restaurant, bar, and sports stadium, has a dependency risk factor of 15 percent, whereas marijuana's is 9 percent.[5] After an adult turns twenty-five, the risk factor for marijuana dependency goes to almost zero.[6] Imagine the number of arrests made and families torn apart owing to the belief that marijuana is a potentially serious addiction problem for adults.

The parents who come to me are making the decision to try cannabis after discovering firsthand the knowns. They've already had to wean their kids off opioids after a sports injury, or sit by them in the hospital as their bodies recuperate from a rare but nearly lethal response to an FDA-approved medication. When I hear about a doctor saying he doesn't know enough about cannabis to recommend it or prescribe it, I always wonder: How can he prescribe a drug that he *does* know is dangerous?

I am a parent, so I can feel my blood begin to boil with frustration on behalf of parents who've lost loved ones because of this irrational stance on medication. My heart breaks for them, but it is not always the doctors' fault. I have many friends and colleagues in the medical field. They are passionate, rational, and mostly overworked. They see too many patients in one day to spend hours researching the effects of the drugs they do prescribe, let alone cannabis. (Some are aware of the medicinal benefits of the plant but fear losing their job if they speak up.) I offer no blame for the gut-wrenching statistic that the third leading cause of death in America is medical error.[7] I offer help. I believe that cannabis, done correctly, will reduce harmful medication and ease the strain on the health field. For parents offered the choice between giving their teens opioids or cannabis for pain, I believe cannabis is the more conservative choice.

Is cannabis harmful to young users? It can be. Is cannabis addiction a problem? Yes. Are candies filled with cannabis that are sold at pot shops worrisome for parents and pet owners? Absolutely. Emergency room visits for overdoses of cannabis have increased in Colorado since legalization of the drug.[8] But these visits do not end in death. Developing and prescribing drugs that can reduce the use of other drugs known to cause fatal overdoses is a no-brainer for a parent.

Cannabis in Utero

Regardless of your view of cannabis, you were essentially born with it coursing through your body. Endocannabinoids are present soon after conception, when stem cells are dividing exponentially. Cannabinoids help regulate this miraculous proliferation of cells.[9] Cannabinoids are also present in breast milk.[10] It is thought that they might help stimulate the baby's appetite.[11] Colloquially, we call this the munchies. In cancer wards, it is called *appetite stimulation* and can be a matter of life or death for patients with wasting syndrome. Cannabinoid-induced appetite stimulation has contributed to the survival of the human species since the dawn of time. Researchers in Israel, who discovered the ECS, are far more advanced in cannabinoid research than in the West. Here is the conclusion of a 2004 study on using cannabinoids to aid in pediatric cancer symptoms, which include lack of appetite: "Excellent clinical results have . . . been reported in pediatric oncology and in case studies of children with severe neurological disease or brain trauma. We suggest cannabinoid treatment for children or young adults with cystic fibrosis in order to achieve an improvement of their health condition including improved food intake and reduced inflammatory exacerbations."[12]

Just because we have endocannabinoids in our body doesn't mean phytocannabinoids are acceptable for babies. But it gives rise to the question, What is acceptable for babies? The subject of pharmaceuticals came up with a friend of mine who is a midwife. I asked her what was given to mothers for pain during childbirth. She mentioned the opioid fentanyl, which I had heard about from a client. (Other drugs containing the active molecule in fentanyl are Sublimaze, Actin, Durogesic, Fentora, Matrifen, Haldid, Onsolis, Instanyl, Abstral, and Lazanda, to name a few.) Given to her for pain relief during cancer treatment, my client neglected to take her dose one night and was wrenched awake in a cold sweat, suffering from painful muscle spasms. She thought she might be having a stroke or heart attack and called her doctor, who said she needed to go back on the fentanyl. Her body was having withdrawal symptoms similar to those caused by heroin. My client was not interested in being addicted to synthetic heroin, so she came to me to learn about medical marijuana. Thus, my impression of fentanyl was that it is not something you'd want to give a pregnant mother or her newborn.

"Wait, they give fentanyl to mothers during childbirth?" I asked the midwife.

"It's not a big deal, really. It's common. It doesn't stay in the bloodstream very long, so its effects are short lived."

To put it in context, fentanyl, a Schedule II drug, is different from morphine, the active molecule derived from the common garden poppy that is processed into heroin (a Schedule I, dangerous drug with no medical benefits, according to the FDA). It is different from morphine in that it is fifty to a hundred times *more potent*.[13] It is on the 2017 World Health Organization's list of "essential medicines, the most effective and safe medicines needed in a health system."[14] According to the United Nations Office on Drugs and

Crime, some analogues of fentanyl have been created that are ten thousand times more potent than morphine.[15] I don't mean to be alarmist. I'm sure millions of babies are born with heroin-times-one-hundred coursing through their bloodstream for a few hours, and they turn out just fine. But there are potential side effects for the mother and baby. Fentanyl can effectively reduce pain and anxiety for the mother. But she may also experience nausea, vomiting, itching, decreased gastric motility, loss of protective airway reflexes, and hypoxia due to respiratory depression.[16] Hypoxia is a deficiency of oxygen in the tissues. The potent opiate also crosses into the placenta.[17] Here are the possible side effects for the newborn baby: central nervous system depression, respiratory depression, impaired early breast-feeding, altered neurological behavior, and decreased ability to regulate body temperature.[18] In one NIH study, fentanyl was recommended as the preferred opiate for childbirth as it was *less* harmful than others. It concluded with the following statement: "Questions remain regarding the neurologic impact of these anesthetics in preterm infants."[19] That phrase sounds a lot like "there's not enough evidence" arguments used against cannabis. It is interesting to note that Insys Therapeutics Inc., a company that makes a type of fentanyl spray used for pain relief, donated $500,000 to fight marijuana legalization efforts in Arizona in 2016.[20]

What might be the ramifications of prescribing cannabis to the mother in the same situation? Cannabinoids can effectively reduce pain[21] and anxiety,[22] so one could make a comparison between the two drugs. Although smoking is not effective in treating many symptoms, an inhaled, vaporous form would enter the mother's lungs and deliver cannabinoids rapidly to her central nervous system through the bloodstream. It is the fastest way to deliver a dose without overdoing it. (If she didn't want it in inhaled form, a sublingual lozenge or tincture might have a similar effect. A suppository at the birth canal or topical on the belly might also be therapeutic.) The inhaled cannabinoids would be activating cells in the upper extremity of the mother first, before circulating through the bloodstream and entering the placenta. Initially, we'd hope the mother would experience the desired reduction of pain and anxiety. Cannabinoids can also decrease blood pressure, as they help dilate capillaries.[23] They have antinausea and antiemetic effects and could prove useful if she also happened to be injected with fentanyl. Cannabinoids could also conceivably *increase* airflow and oxygen to tissues, as they dilate blood vessels in the lungs. Similarly to the opioid, cannabinoids can reduce gastric motility, but this may be a good thing for moms pushing a baby out of their nether regions. Cannabinoids primarily function as regulators, so the motility of the intestines could be properly regulated instead of reduced. Cannabis is not known to cause constipation,[24] but opiates can.[25]

The baby will also presumably receive some of these cannabinoids. Cannabinoids can relax muscles and decrease anxiety, but they do not dangerously depress the central nervous system because we have cannabinoid receptors all over the body. Opiate receptors are located in an important spot in the brain—the spot that keeps us breathing. Since cannabinoids are part of the natural breast-feeding process, these phytocannabinoids may encourage early breast-feeding in the infant. As far as the effect on neurological behavior, as with the fentanyl, it is difficult to say clinically what the cannabinoids would do to the infant's brain. There is no definitive evidence that cannabinoids have long-term neurological effects on the human brain. According to the study out of Israel mentioned earlier, the endocannabinoid nearly identical to THC, anandamide, "protects the developing brain from trauma-induced neuronal loss."[26]

Another perception often perpetuated by the medical field is the correlation between mothers who smoke marijuana and their baby's low birth weight.[27] It is general knowledge that alcohol and caffeine are to be avoided during pregnancy due to their correlation to low birth weight as well. (Incidentally, both are legal.) But some of the more widely referenced studies pertaining to cannabis and low birthweight are neither definitive nor particularly illuminating. One concludes that "the relationship was observed only among European-American mothers, but not in mothers of different ethnicities."[28] Another concludes, "This study found lower birth weight for infants exposed to cannabis when exposure was measured with urine testing, but not when exposure was self-reported."[29] Another found that "one meta-analysis established that frequent cannabis use (4 or more times a week) was related to a decrease in mean birth weight. However, the overall pooled estimate of low birth weights was not significant."[30]

I'm not suggesting that mothers should smoke cannabis if there is no medical need, but as with many of the medical claims of the harm done by cannabis, there is evidence to the contrary. Much of it is a correlation at best but can be erroneously spread as scientific fact by the medical community and those who report on the studies.

One ethnographic study conducted by Dr. Melanie Dreher found no such correlation, let alone causation, between low birth weight and cannabis in her research on Jamaican pregnant mothers who smoked during pregnancy.[31] The researcher expected to find low birth weight or neurological issues in the babies whose mothers smoked on a daily basis. But as is the case with many in-depth studies related to cannabis, she found evidence for the opposite effect. The babies were more regulated than the babies born of mothers who did not smoke cannabis. She found the babies to be more socially responsive, more stable autonomically, and they had better self-regulation. In the researcher's words, "It does not seem to make a difference in the productivity of the people in Jamaica [and] it seems to make no difference in terms of exposure during pregnancy. . . . We looked at these children again at age five, both groups of children, and could find absolutely nothing that linked their development with their exposure during pregnancy."[32]

When you have a basic understanding of the importance of the endocannabinoid system, this outcome is not so shocking. What becomes counterintuitive is the theory that a chemical known for aiding in the proliferation of stem cells would ultimately cause low birth weight. These outcomes were comparing infants born of Jamaican mothers who did not smoke at all and Jamaican mothers who had a religious and daily connection to the herb. These daily users are what I would call chronic users.

Unless the medical need outweighs the potential risks, it is not necessary for pregnant women to smoke daily. But certainly they should not be prosecuted nor shamed for using cannabis to reduce nausea, pain, anxiety, or other disorders, when the readily available drugs doctors *do* prescribe can have measurable negative effects on the fetus and mother. A puff of cannabis or a few drops of tincture during a particularly difficult bout of morning sickness or labor might be a reasonable alternative to a prescription pharmaceutical.

Going back to our birth scenario, there is no evidence whatsoever that a single dose of cannabis (especially after penetrating the placenta) has any adverse long-term effect on the infant brain. If cannabis was called something else and was available as a pain-killing inhalant to laboring mothers, perhaps it would be a reasonable painkiller option, before moving on to a more serious drug such as fentanyl.

Despite the lack of evidence definitively linking cannabis to birth defects, I do know that if THC is found in the blood of the mother or her newborn infant, it is mandated in the United States that health practitioners contact child protective services. Clinical evidence to support this mandate is not in the DEA's favor. Although there are several National Institute of Drug Abuse studies purporting a *correlation* between prenatal marijuana exposure and negative cognitive outcomes in children, many of the studies have been criticized as controlling for factors that seek only the negative outcome. Most were based on data collected from mothers who admitted they smoked marijuana. They tend to be women from lower socioeconomic backgrounds. My assessment is that if a mother is smoking marijuana daily during pregnancy, she may be treating an ailment such as depression that needs to be objectively addressed by a physician. Because the debate is not settled, caution is warranted. An extensive 2017 report compiling the data since 1999 does find statistical evidence correlating lower birth weight and cannabis use, but this does not automatically imply harm. The report concludes, "There is insufficient evidence to support or refute a statistical association between maternal cannabis smoking and later outcomes in the offspring (e.g., sudden infant death syndrome, cognition/academic achievement, and later substance use)."[33] Apparently, cannabis-using mothers are neglecting their children, but scientifically speaking, we're not sure how. It is clear that new studies need to be performed by objective researchers with our current scientific and cultural understanding in mind.

I do not scorn the medical practitioners, or the mothers who opt for highly potent opioids during childbirth. But this is a discussion about a single medication. Dozens of other drugs are given to pregnant and nursing mothers for nausea, pain, anxiety, depression, allergies, colds, and other ailments. There's even a name for drugs that harm babies during pregnancy: teratogens. Some antidepressants, anticonvulsants, antibiotics, anticoagulants, and some blood pressure medications are known teratogens.[34] Many of these FDA-approved drugs work wonders, but not all of them work for everyone. That is why pharmaceutical companies keep producing more options to treat various ailments. Cannabinoids are merely another option, and they are produced by our body, from the moment of conception until the day we die. Patients and practitioners ultimately have to do what is comfortable for them. But just because the FDA gives drugs the go-ahead doesn't mean they are not harmful—or even less harmful than a plant that mimics the chemicals we already produce in our bodies.

One can thus empathize with the dilemma a parent faces in deciding whether to use conventional drugs they know are harming their child versus one that brings relief but puts the parent in legal jeopardy.

Toddlers

Simon was a charming and social two-year-old. When his mom brought him to my home office for a cannabis consultation, he crawled off the couch, hobbled over to where I was sitting, and proceeded to enjoy the entire session from my lap. He was happy, but he was not well. Simon had been born with a form of epilepsy that caused dozens of seizures per day. His young parents had witnessed these daily seizures, but they had also witnessed the effect of the medication prescribed to control them. The class of drugs available to treat seizures and convulsions is a powerful one. Often the seizures outweigh the debilitating side effects, but for Simon it was a tossup. He was curious, joyful, and active with no medication, but his seizures were incapacitating. On medication, his seizures were reduced but he was a zombie. Listless and sedated, Simon would sleep all day long.

His parents had gone through many different drugs to find a balance, with little success. When they watched a CNN segment about a little girl named Charlotte whose parents reduced her seizures by using a particular strain of cannabis,[35] they wanted more answers. It took them months to find a pediatrician who was not dismissive of their questions about medical cannabis. Eventually, they did find a doctor who supported their efforts, but he had no authority to prescribe it and little information about how they would go about utilizing it.

After learning about Simon and the drugs he'd tried, I eased into the conversation about giving cannabis to him. I was growing strains high in

THC, a strain purportedly high in CBD as well, and I also had pure CBD oil. Although Simon's mom was open to anything at this point, his dad was scared of yet another drug, especially an illegal one. I empathized with his fears and told him that there was a way to introduce it gently to the body without Simon ingesting it or experiencing psychotropic effects.

"Research shows that CBD and THC are more effective if they work together in what's called an 'entourage effect.' But I think the high CBD strain I grow might still be too strong in THC for him. If we can get good results without the THC, then all the better. What I recommend is starting with a CBD concentrate infused in olive oil."

"But how do we know how much he should take?" Asked the dad.

"I would avoid having him ingest it at all. Since his seizures are nerve related, I would suggest the CBD be applied topically first."

"But what is applying it to his skin going to do?" He asked impatiently.

"I know it seems strange, but we're trying to give him as small a dose as we possibly can and then increase it. He can take the oil internally, but I would suggest taking just a few drops of oil and massaging it into the base of his neck and continue down the spine and out to his limbs. It may be difficult to see results right away. It could take a month for oils to penetrate all the tissue layers.[36] We don't really address this massage method in conventional medicine, so there's no scientific study to back that up. But the hope is that it can get into his nerves all over his body and regulate the over-firing that is occurring." At this point I felt like a snake-oil salesman. I had no idea whether it would work, and I was telling them it *wouldn't* until they'd probably exhausted their bottle of oil and needed another one. Although it's a nice marketing technique, I was far more interested in positive results than in selling a useless bottle of oil.

The mom wanted to take the CBD oil as well as the THC oil I made because she too had heard they work better together. But the dad vetoed the idea. They left with a small bottle of CBD oil. After a couple weeks I called them to see if there was any progress.

"It's really hard to tell if it's working." Said Simon's mom. To me that meant there had been no positive results.

"How are you using it?" I asked.

"Well, we put a couple drops into yogurt and he eats it. He still has about six to ten small seizures a day, though."

"Sounds like little progress. Have you tried applying it topically at all?" I asked.

"Well, we haven't really done that. It just seems sort of weird to put it on his skin, but I'm giving him a bath tonight so I can try it a little," she said.

"I know it's weird, but maybe this will help to just give it a shot. I like to emphasize medicated oil massage to caretakers because we get so caught up in the treatments that we forget the deeper connection between caretaker and patient. In Sanskrit, the word 'oil' is the same for the word 'love.' So regardless of whether the CBD oil works, maybe you can think of it as just giving him some loving touch—a little oil massage before his bath. You can put a few drops in a regular massage oil to make the CBD last longer."

The idea seemed reasonable, so she gave it a shot. A week later she came back again, this time for the oil that contained THC. She still wasn't sure if the CBD oil itself was working, but the oil massages seemed to be helping him. I watched many clients go through this logic. Sometimes my suggestion was so mild that they wanted a stronger remedy just so they could see the results. THC is a powerful compound, so if you take enough, you can feel or observe the effect. This is a plus if you're a caregiver working with a patient who may not be able to verbalize the outcome. The patient will essentially become stoned with a high dose of THC, making the effect observable. "Stoned" is a crass word to apply to a toddler with epilepsy, but remember, we're talking about results, not perception. We didn't want Simon stoned, but perhaps we did want his frenetic nerves to be stoned.

I talked to Simon's mom a few weeks later, and she was upbeat. Simon was doing better. She didn't know if it was because of the oil or not. Her prebath ritual of putting the oil on his body felt good to both of them. She was more connected, and he enjoyed the "love" he was getting. He had fully weaned himself from all pharmaceuticals, and mom noticed a reduction in the number and duration of his seizures. I knew the oil penetrating his skin every night wasn't hurting him. I also knew that the science behind the cannabinoids could back up some positive results. She was thrilled.

"He's not on any of the drugs that turned him into a zombie. We managed to wean him off all of them, actually. He's developing somewhat normally now. Before, he wasn't moving at all. He wasn't alert. Not being on all that junk is just so relieving."

I came away wondering if my cannabis products were actually helping. It was a trial of one subject, after all. Although scientific trials can be flawed and rarely measure things like *love,* I do like to have a scientific foundation for treatment. But Simon's mom was less stressed, and he was thriving. In her eyes, he was being helped. According to science, we were introducing a chemical to his body that it was familiar with—that it used to regulate nerve behavior. In the eyes of the law, however, I was distributing a Schedule I substance to a minor.

There are now organizations devoted to educating parents about the benefits of medical cannabis for children. Many of them are formed when a parent, unable to find relief through conventional methods, discovers that cannabis can help. A miraculous recovery ensues, and the parents become advocates. They are not stoners or hippies. They are concerned parents merely looking for options. These outcomes are reminding parents that there are benefits to utilizing the full spectrum of medicine—from herbal home remedies to the more powerful THC-filled cannabis, to the technology that contemporary medicine has to offer.

Preteens

I am grateful that both my children made it through their toddler years without any serious medical issues. But by the time my daughter was about four years old, she was following me into the basement to watch me water my plants. The image of a child helping her dad in his cannabis garden is a shocking one. Before she became utterly bored with my medical marijuana and gardening obsession a couple of years later, she saw what looked like fun and wanted to help. Unlike a neighbor of mine, who has never revealed her growing passion to her nine-year-old son, I chose not to hide it. Perhaps what I was cultivating was illegal, but it wasn't wrong. What's the harm in letting her pour water into a potted plant or cut dead leaves off with scissors, I rationalized? We never uttered the words "marijuana" or "cannabis" in the house until it was my public profession. We often referred to my operation as "the basement garden" or "daddy's plants." Being a science teacher and concerned parent, I knew there was nothing intrinsically immoral or unsafe with her helping me. She wasn't getting high down there and neither was I. She wasn't even touching the plants. The pleasure she derived was the same that anyone gets looking at a lush garden in the middle of winter. But she got to share the experience with me.

Like many closeted growers, I wanted to share my love for the underground growing process with anyone, including my daughter. At the time, the journalist Andrew Sullivan had a popular online blog called "The Dish" where he published an anonymous, reader-contributed book called *The Cannabis Closet*. It was with great pride that I submitted the following letter and was included in the publication:

A Reader Writes:

I am a high school teacher and married with two children in Massachusetts. I also grow a small amount of Marijuana (six plants on average). During harvest time, the basement is abustle with trimming.

My four-year-old daughter, who loves gardening and always asks to help, is allowed to cut the large leaves from the plants. She asks questions about trimming and the flowers, about the seeds, why we hang it upside down when we dry it, etc. I answer honestly.

I have been easing my daughter into the "some people believe it is harmful, so they don't want me to have it," conversation, which she listens to without judgment. But we never name it. It's always, "the plants," or "medicine." Any other terminology is like profanity for my kids. If they know the word, they may utter it in an inappropriate place.

My high school students, who are "from the hood," are completely out of the cannabis closet—a cultural phenomenon I believe contributes to the disparity between white and minority drug arrests. Despite the fact that I am outspoken about legalization, and that "I too smoked some weed in college," they have no idea about my current relationship with the drug. How I wish I could create a school marijuana garden to create the same interest, curiosity, and patience in my troubled students that my daughter experiences in our year-round garden.

I was proud. I was revealing to the world, albeit anonymously, that as a middle-class, law-abiding adult, I had a beloved cannabis garden. I was a doting father. I wanted to share my knowledge and help alter the economics of the inner city and the imbalance in the justice system. I was altruistic and trusting.

Unfortunately, my vision was too far advanced for even those still in the closet. The next letter in the book reads as follows:

A Reader Writes:

Hey man, you gotta call that cat out. Nobody should be allowing a four year old to help in the trimming of weed. I understand it's not a lot of weed, and I'm a huge stoner, and whatever. My old man grows a small batch of herb for himself and whatever. I get it. Weed's not that bad. But YOUR FOUR YEAR OLD? That's just not cool.

I know marijuana is decriminalized in Massachusetts, but it's still illegal, especially to grow. And this is an ADULT product, like alcohol. That's the argument we're all trying to make here. Massholes like this are the reason people say stoners are criminals.

"Masshole" is a derogatory slang term for a Massachusett's resident.

Despite my fatherly approach, my wife put a stop to it. To this day, revealing my children's knowledge of my illicit garden is the aspect of my marijuana journey that is the most difficult for her to reveal to others. I understand the concern. We don't want people to think we're bad parents, that we would do something blithe and dangerous. The war on drugs failed, I often say. But the government has won many of its battles. Instilling deep paranoia and irrational fear in billions of people worldwide is one of them. An adult is growing six organic marijuana plants, while thousands of people are slaughtered every year by drug cartels in Mexico. Wasn't I providing a safer alternative? Prescription drugs and legal alcohol kill thousands of children a year in America. There is no evidence, other than the legal ramifications of being deemed negligent, that I was neglecting my child. In hindsight, I realized the legal risk that I was putting my children in was substantial. When I was raided, by far the most traumatic facet was the investigation of possible child neglect by the Department of Children and Families.

I knew my rationale would not hold up in court. If I were a wine maker and my four-year-old smashed grapes, would I be deemed negligent? If I brewed beer in my basement and allowed a four-year-old to measure out ingredients—or God forbid, taste the bitter result—would I be deemed a criminal neglecting my child?

Cannabis was illegal. I got it. I was perhaps naive. But it was the twenty-first century, and the conversation about cannabis was and still is steeped in fear and irrationality. Did my white privilege make me believe I wouldn't get caught, that a prosecution wouldn't rip our family apart as it does for others, Caucasians included? Yes. But it was also my belief in the difference between right and wrong. It's wrong to be a stoner. It's wrong to not pursue the facts. It's wrong to hide your cannabis because of guilt and shame. If you're ashamed about being an addict, get help. But don't be ashamed that you regulate your body chemistry with a natural medicine over a synthetic one.

Cannabis users are the brunt of jokes and stereotyping in film and media. We roll our eyes at pot culture, but it is called a drug war for a reason. Laugh at stoners all you want. There are children who are safe and feel loved by their parents that are being dragged away from them by authorities. It is a battleground the government still controls.

Fighting fear with rationality requires discipline. I was a trusting father, but I wasn't stupid. I walked my daughter through "the conversation" early on and many times as she and her brother got older.

"Honey, I want to explain something about my plants to you," I would begin.

"Your plants?" she asked.

"You know, my plants down in the basement."

"Oh, right. What about them?"

"First, I want you to know that I would never do anything to hurt you or the family. I grow those plants and you can see that they are not hurting us. It is a plant. It is a plant that has been a medicine for thousands of years, but there are some people who believe this plant can be dangerous and some people have decided that it should be illegal."

"Illegal? But it's just a plant?" she said.

"Yes, I know it's confusing. But it means that if the police saw that I was growing this plant, they would not like it. They would take the plant away and I'd get in trouble," I explained.

My daughter was mature for her age. Legal issues were complicated, but we were friendly with the police who ate at the diner we frequented. She understood their authority and she understood right and wrong. She could understand the difference between a plant I grew in our home and violence, for example.

"Dangerous? But it's just a plant!? I don't understand why it's bad," she wondered. It was the politics that were difficult to explain.

"Well, you know how alcohol is something that only adults can drink, and we don't let kids drink alcohol?"

"Yeah."

"Well, this plant is like that. It is only for adults to use and it's not appropriate for kids. (I avoided the medical argument to keep it simple.) Some people drink a lot of alcohol, and they can get sick because it can be poisonous. They can even die. Especially kids." I said.

"Can you die from your plants? Are they poisonous?" she asked.

"No, you can't. No one has ever died directly from the plants I grow. But you can feel sick from having too much of it. Or you can be unhealthy if you use it too much. So we have to be careful how we use it. It is not a dangerous plant if used appropriately. I would never bring a plant or something into the home that would be dangerous to you or your baby brother."

I was glad she didn't ask why alcohol was legal *and* poisonous. Child alcohol poisonings account for about four thousand fatalities a year in the United States.[37] The subject would be difficult and scary for her. Marijuana discussion is not alarming if you remove irrational paranoia from the equation.

The conversation should have been more difficult. It encouraged me to question what actually was dangerous in my home. Cannabis is a proven anti-inflammatory and analgesic, so I researched the toxicity of household painkillers as a comparison. An Internet search revealed to me that nonsteroidal anti-inflammatory drugs (NSAIDS), such as ibuprofen, are responsible for tens of thousands of emergency-room visits a year.[38] How horrible is that, I thought. Cough syrup is another danger. According to the National Institute of Drug Abuse, "When taken in high doses, [over-the-counter cough medicine] acts on the same cell receptors as dissociative hallucinogenic drugs like

PCP."[39] We specifically give these drugs to children. They're fine in low doses, like cannabis, but they can be abused, also like cannabis. I saw the double standard, and I let go of allowing my daughter to help. But I began storing over-the-counter drugs farther out of reach. It seems that drug education is neither objective nor particularly helpful in keeping kids safe.

Several years later, after a long day of writing for this book, I tucked my ten-year-old daughter into bed. I lingered, because even though I felt passionate about educating and providing patients with medical marijuana, I knew she saw a different side to it. As she developed, the conversation would have to develop as well. She didn't pore over the scientific studies the way I did. But she did experience the fallout from police raiding our home. And she knew I had more than just a professional relationship with it. Sometimes she would come outside when I had finished smoking from a little water pipe. The pipe would be sitting on the deck next to me. She didn't question it or criticize me, but I worried that I was sending her mixed messages. I didn't have a debilitating disease. I smoked cannabis much the way one would use red wine at the end of the day. Adults generally know red wine is helpful for heart health, but let's face it: most of us are putting our feet up and using it to take the edge off. I waited until she settled into bed and then I took on a serious tone.

"I know you understand how medical marijuana is used, but what do you really think about the fact that I smoke marijuana?" I'd never used that phrase before with my kids. We had avoided charged phrases for a good reason. At a flea market when she was five years old, she saw a pot leaf necklace and proclaimed with excitement, "There's Dad's plant!" Despite our openness at home, we knew how easily she could give us away. At ten, it seemed appropriate to have a deeper conversation about its grittier side. I awaited her answer with trepidation, but she didn't skip a beat.

"I know it will never kill you, so I'm okay with it," she said.

That put everything in perspective for me. In her eyes, the most important requirement was that her parents stay alive. Of all the harms associated with cannabis—accurately or otherwise—fatality was not one of them. The same could not be said of alcohol, many over-the-counter pills, and prescription drugs. For a preteen trying to make sense of the world through the actions of her parents, moderate cannabis use was acceptable. She saw us go to work every day, put food on the table, tuck her into bed. Her life was stable, and cannabis didn't register as something that took us away from her.

We live in a culture swayed by the perception of cannabis. I have seen adults give sips of wine to their children in restaurants. Disease and accidents associated with alcohol make it the fourth leading cause of death in the United States,[40] but if we let a child try cannabis, we are the vilest of parents. We have a fear that loss of cognition—being high—is not only a scourge on society but a slippery slope for children. Perhaps we fear that after one toke they will embrace altered consciousness like a mouse tapping a lever that delivers a constant stream of crack cocaine, never to return again. When we give a sip of wine to our child in a restaurant or at Thanksgiving dinner, we are aware of its dangers, but we do not set out to get them drunk. It is difficult to "sip" cannabis. If humans succumb to the addiction of altered consciousness, it is worrisome. Abuse of illegal drugs, prescription medicine, sex, shopping, sugar, video games, exercise, and risky behavior is all harmful. But abuse is the problem. Moderate use is not. I do not want my daughter to be traumatized by my cannabis use or think I'm hiding some shameful crime. I want her to be aware of how and why I use it, so that she can see a model of use that is appropriate, adult, and safe. When I am on my smart phone too much, she chastises me for it and I put it away. If I'm always smoking pot, she should feel comfortable calling me out in that regard as well. Being open in the household about boundaries and potential addiction keeps my family in check.

The preteen years are an appropriate time to speak to your children about cannabis. If they are already dealing with trauma, abuse, or neglect, it may be too late. The pull of cannabis to alleviate these issues is great, and they may be self-medicating or abusing it already. If they are physically and emotionally stable, then they are old enough to understand why an adult might use it. And they are probably young enough to avoid using it themselves. Many parents attempt to have the conversation when their children are in their midteens, long after their kids have been exposed to it at parties, via older friends, or by another relative. By then, kids know it is something to keep secret. If the parents approach the subject with fear or judgment, the secret will be kept. With the additional burden of shame, guilt, and secrecy, the pot stash will find a deeper hiding place in the closet or dresser. Keeping marijuana out of the hands of children has little to do with regulations requiring dispensaries to sell products in child-proof containers or the number of feet from a school the store fronts are allowed to conduct business. These regulations give a false sense of security to parents. My ten-year-old daughter will be more equipped to understand the dangers and pitfalls of teen cannabis abuse because I know the facts and I am open and honest about using it.

The Challenge of Cannabis Edibles

The conversation around appropriate cannabis use is generally straightforward in my household. My children are still young, and by now they have been driven to boredom enough times by my lectures on the subject that they avoid it at all costs. Not so with sugary treats. In my early days of rediscovering cannabis, I used to make pot brownies, but then my kids got old enough to recognize a delicious treat when they saw one. I knew a brownie wasn't going to shut down my kids' organs, but why risk having them nab one? It is also important to keep in mind that if we're staying true to our health, we might ask ourselves whether candy or sugar treats are the best medium for delivering medicinal cannabis to the body. If cannabis edibles are unsweetened and boring to the young palate, it reduces the likelihood that children will try them, let alone overdose on them.

There are also two basic reasons why sugar and cannabis are an inappropriate combination. For one, sugary treats are extremely delicious. When was the last time you opened a bag of M&Ms or gummy bears and ate precisely one? If you're like me, you rationalize eating the entire bag so that they will not tempt you anymore. As many adults, kids, and pets have discovered, this is a very scary scenario for treats infused with cannabis. A dispensary can put all the warning information it wants on the side of a package of cannabis edibles. But it will not determine precisely how it will affect the patient or inadvertent user. Chocolate bars, gummies, and cannabis soda do not lend themselves to a conservative approach to medicating. For thousands of years, humans have been trying to get as much sugar and fat into their systems as possible—just in case the mastodon herd or wild blueberry harvest doesn't come back next season. If your appropriate dose of cannabis to treat your symptoms is one gummy bear, then you might as well take a couple drops of tincture or oil. Go buy a bag of conventional gummy bears if you must have them. But that leads to the second reason why cannabis and sugar are not a healthy mix: it has been well established that glucose feeds cancer cells[41] and exacerbates inflammation.[42]

To apply the cannabis candy scenario to a house with children in it is asking for trouble. Marijuana dispensaries in Massachusetts have razor wire around their grow facility perimeters. They have armed guards at entrances who check IDs. Surveillance cameras project ID images on screens inside the building before a patient is allowed to be buzzed in to the facility. These regulations are imposed to prevent the diversion of marijuana to children (and adults without medical marijuana licenses). But the moment a patient walks out of the dispensary with his delicious cannabis chocolates, these regulations are useless. There is no easy way to stop the cannabis from getting into the body of a kid or pet. A label stating "Keep out of reach of children" on a candy bar is laughable to a parent of an eight-year-old. In my home, we already keep noncannabis treats out of reach of our children. Yet my children have shown themselves to be quite resourceful at accessing the treats over the years.

Pets and children overdosing—taking an uncomfortable amount—of edible cannabis is already happening in Colorado and other states where edibles are readily sold in stores. Overdoses have caused cannabis-related emergency room visits to increase substantially.[43] Because accidental prescription drug ingestion causes fatalities in children and pets, I still maintain that the cannabis products are less harmful overall. But with new methods of making cannabis stronger, small children and pets can have dangerous responses to the drug. A traditional approach of sugar-free and whole cannabis products is a safer approach. It is not an issue that will be fully resolved. Even experienced adults can take too much and find themselves in a miserable state for many hours. One of my early clients who suffered a frightful cannabis overdose was a middle-aged mom looking to combat her depression and sleeplessness. She had never tried cannabis in any form. I cooked a batch of coconut oil with sativa strains of cannabis—those containing stimulating cannabinoids—and suggested she take a small amount of oil internally. Then, she should wait an hour to feel the effects. (My new recommendation is to wait a full twenty-four hours before increasing the dose.) I hoped the outcome would be a bright, uplifting high to snap her out of her depression. The printed label on the jar said "start with a half teaspoon," but I crossed it out and wrote "*quarter* teaspoon" instead, just to be safe. Looking back, I don't feel I spent enough time getting to know her or the context of her depression. Perhaps if I had, I would have made it very clear what the outcome could be if she thought a bigger dose correlated with a magical reversal of symptoms. I had seen some clients be lifted out of a depressive state with certain sativa strains. Their creativity and joy come back, and they feel inspired to move their bodies and be in nature. But the dose, as well as the experience, has to be presented correctly.

I sent my client on her way. A few days later, I got an angry text from her adult daughter telling me her mother had eaten my oil and was probably having a heart attack. She said she had called the paramedics and they wanted to talk to me. Before I was able to pick my jaw up, the phone started ringing. I was in the middle of washing dishes while my family lounged around the adjacent living room. I wiped my hands, calmly walked out the back door, and picked up the phone. I assumed this was my last hour of freedom. Perhaps the police were already on their way to my house.

"Hello, this is Ezra." Should I sound professional or contrite?

"Are you the person who created this uh, sa-tie-vuh oil? There's a woman here who has an extremely elevated heart rate and we may need to take her to the hospital." He didn't seem accusatory, but there was some panic in his voice.

"Uh, okay. Yes, So I am a medical marijuana consultant and that is oil-infused medical cannabis." How useless my words seemed! My heart was beating in my throat.

"We're trying to determine how much she took and whether it could be life threatening. She says she took two spoonfuls of the oil."

"Oh, no! Two *spoonfuls?* That's not good. She's taken way too much. I thought I had written on the label that she should take a much smaller dose." I immediately felt as if I had failed—with my client and with my impending trial. I was admitting that I gave it to her.

I had researched cannabis-induced fatality at length. I knew no direct fatality had been recorded. But I wasn't the trained paramedic at the scene. In that moment, I wondered if I would truly be the first person in recorded history to have delivered a fatal dose of cannabis.

"Yeah, she clearly took more than that. It's written right here on the bottle to take a quarter teaspoon and wait an hour—hey, Bob, ask her if she waited an hour after her first dose—yeah, she says she waited an hour and nothing happened, so she took another full spoonful. So what's going to happen? I'm trying to determine if she needs to go to the ER or not."

The paramedic was turning to me for medical advice. I was speechless. I assumed his next call was to the police, but he wanted my professional prognosis. Five minutes ago, I was scrubbing dishes. Now I was triaging a potential heart attack victim after a 911 call.

"Um—well, I have to defer to your medical expertise, sir. I do know that the only ingredients in that are the coconut oil and cannabis. No one has ever directly—uh—died from cannabis. I'm pretty confident she'll be okay. But you should—uh—take her to the hospital if you feel her situation is life threatening."

"She's pretty bad. She has an extremely elevated heart rate—into the range of stroke-inducing. She's saying she feels like she's going to die. I think she should probably go to the ER. But you need to tell me if you think she's going to be okay or whether we should take her in."

"Uh—well then, yes, I think you should take her in. I think she's going to survive, but you're the paramedic. If you think she may be in danger of a stroke, then I think she should probably go to the hospital." The situation was too serious to care about keeping myself out of jail. As I paced on my back porch in my socks, what seemed most important was preserving her life. I would suffer the consequences later.

Within minutes of hanging up, my fight-or-flight reaction settled down and my rational mind came back online. I was 100 percent certain that even eight times the recommended dose of cannabis was not going to kill my client. She was not going to have a heart attack or stroke. In hindsight, I could have saved her a lot of trouble—and embarrassment—if I had taken charge over the telephone. When she and I debriefed over the phone a few days later, I got the impression that part of her depression came from her unsympathetic daughter and her social isolation. The flashing lights of the ambulance, her daughter calling 911, and even the paramedic's feeling out of control were exacerbating her cannabis-induced panic attack. What she needed was professional guidance and empathy. If I could have done it over again, I would have asked to speak with her. With the most measured, confident, and compassionate voice I could muster, I would have told her that she was not going to die. I would have told her that she just took too much and what she was experiencing was terrifying but completely normal. She should get comfortable, reduce stimuli in the room, and take deep breaths. If she could eat, oil-rich food like peanut butter would help absorb the THC. The terpene α-pinene, often found in indica or sedative cannabis varieties (and pine forests worldwide), has been shown to induce physiological relaxation and significantly decrease heart rate.[44] A few deep inhalations of a sandal wood candle, cedar moth balls, or pine branch could have made the difference for her. A high dose of CBD may have helped as well, but it would be difficult to convince a person in that state to consume more cannabis.

She was upset and would probably never get to experience the joyous inspiration of a proper dose of cannabis. I was just glad she was alive. I wondered how many doctors had had to answer a similar call for a drug they prescribed. How many of their patients could survive an eightfold dose?

We can put cherry-flavored liquor in the centers of gourmet chocolate (or cover espresso beans with chocolate), but a large number of them would have to be eaten for a person to get drunk, let alone feel she needed to go to the emergency room. Cannabis is less toxic but has far more power by volume than alcohol. In time, with the guidance of educated professionals who know and care about the clients they serve, the public will understand both the power and relative safety of cannabis edibles. Legalizing cannabis edibles means they will be regulated, free of unknown ingredients, and more consistent. If the cannabis is causing a reduction in potentially fatal pharmaceuticals, then even these powerful edibles are creating a net safety benefit in the home. Although there have been some reports of cannabis edibles correlated with fatalities in Colorado,[45] the likelihood that a fatal amount of raw cannabis product would be ingested is extremely low. Raw cannabis doesn't taste very good. A human would have to eat many pounds of concentrated cannabis resin to reach the levels tested in large animals, levels that still failed to result in fatality.

If legislatures are concerned about curtailing the number of marijuana overdoses, they should leave production of cannabis sugar products up to consumers. Dispensaries would be let mostly off the hook when it came to accidental ingestion if they were able to sell only nonsugar products. If college kids want Jell-O shots, they have to make them on their own. Cannabis candy consumers are just as capable. It's baffling that Colorado allowed all manner of candies, sodas, and other products that look like store-bought candies in its first year of legalization. (Since edibles account for 45 percent of Colorado's pot sales,[46] they are here to stay.) As my case studies demonstrate, cannabis-infused oils and tinctures are just as effective for patients—and can also get you high, if that's your preference. They are neither attractive nor palatable to children. I don't want to disparage the hard-working business owners churning out candy products or the patients who benefit from them, but perhaps individuals and not shops should be responsible for the consequences of the overdoses. I realize this does not solve the issue entirely, but until the populace is educated about how to use cannabis and what it can do to pets and kids, a more conservative (or at least healthy) regulation of edibles as states roll out new marijuana laws is an easy solution.

four

Young Adults

So grand a result, so tiny a sin.

REPORT OF THE INDIAN HEMP DRUGS COMMISSION | 1893–94

Here is a letter of support I received from the parent of a teen:

To the District Attorney,

I am writing this letter to let you know how much Ezra has helped my family. We have consulted with Ezra on several occasions for help with our son who suffers from social anxiety and depression. My son was prescribed medical marijuana by a medical doctor to ease his anxiety and depression. Ezra was extremely helpful and knowledgeable about how best to use cannabis in a way that helped my son's symptoms in a therapeutic way.

I was very surprised when Ezra explained that cannabis could actually exacerbate some of my son's symptoms and that it would be a good idea for him to take a break and stop using the cannabis for a while. This really showed how much Ezra cares for his clients and how passionate he is about cannabis being used appropriately and effectively.

Ezra went out of his way to spend time with us, and as a mom, this meant a lot to me. I can't tell you how many "professionals" we have seen that never seemed to really care about the outcome for my son.

Ezra is an extremely intelligent, passionate, and caring consultant who goes above and beyond to educate his clients in an ethical and supportive manner. I can't tell you how much our family has appreciated his help. Please feel free to contact me if I can help in any other way with his legal case.

Sincerely,
Judy Fowler

Teens

The conversation around teenagers and cannabis use is a loaded one. But as someone who thrives in the gray area between science and subjectivity, I love to have this conversation. Teen cannabis use also illuminates the ignorance on both sides of the debate. The federal stance, via the DEA, is similar to an abstinence-only sex-education platform. Abstinence education has no measurable efficacy and does little to prepare teenagers for the real pitfalls of sex or marijuana.[1] The DEA maintains that decriminalization and legalization will increase teen pot use, but they don't have much clinical evidence to back it up. In fact, evidence shows the opposite. According to a study published in *Child and Adolescent Psychiatry* in 2016,[2] and another in the *Lancet* in 2015,[3] marijuana use among teens has declined in the last decade, despite the advent of widespread decriminalization and legalization laws. Millions of teenagers are therefore deeply skeptical of the authorities who perpetuate this stance.

In addition, because of evolving medical marijuana laws, teens can now call their pot smoking medicinal. Some teenagers are high twenty-four hours a day. Science can't prove definitively that they're damaging their brains, but we have a gut feeling that something isn't right. I know teens who could reduce dangerous alcohol use and risky behavior if they chose cannabis over binge drinking. And I know teens who are stuck in the foggy, feel-good rut that cannabis can dig insidiously into their lives. But they don't want to hear what their parents have to say, especially if it is the party line. Some parents are pro-marijuana use for patients and adults but worry that their teens are in trouble. They want to help but can't reach their teen through the cloud of self-righteousness and addiction.

It may take years for society to come to terms with the reality that close to a third of high school kids have smoked pot recently.[4] Although alcohol use is still more prevalent among teenagers, marijuana can be acquired easily.[5] The disparity between widespread teen use and how to respond to it is ironic. No federally funded school can have a conversation about cannabis that supports anything but complete abstinence for teens or adults. As of this writing, medical marijuana is legal in well over half of U.S. states and the District of Columbia, yet there is no school professional trained to monitor appropriate cannabis use or advise students on how to respond to relatives who are using it legally. In states such as Colorado, the conversation is being forced upon the schools. After a widely publicized case involving a teen medical marijuana user, it is now legal for medical marijuana patients to take medicinal cannabis on school grounds (as long as it is not inhaled),[6] creating headaches for administrators.[7]

The full spectrum needs to be addressed. There are teens who can legitimately benefit from cannabis and there are teens already medicating with cannabis, albeit illegally. There are also teens abusing the drug and for whom abuse is leading them astray from their studies, their families, and their grip on reality. Finally, there are stable teens who are just using it recreationally, albeit illegally. They are good students from stable homes, and they smoke on the weekends. Since the debate about its effect on the brain is unsettled, the most conservative stance is to avoid cannabis altogether until late in one's twenties, when the brain is fully developed. Avoiding sex until marriage is a safe bet too, but good luck convincing a teen of this rationale. Regardless, millions of productive adults have survived smoking occasionally throughout their teens and early twenties. Falling off a bicycle can give you brain damage. Smoking marijuana occasionally isn't even correlated with brain damage. The most dangerous consequences teens face are the justice system (more so if they are poor or belong to a minority) or the wrath of their parents. If they don't get caught or if their parents are informed and communicative, the kids are probably going to be all right. Like the majority of alcohol-drinking adults, they will not abuse the drug into adulthood.

I will address teen cannabis use first from a medicinal perspective. Teenagers with debilitating illnesses, who have found conventional drugs lacking, could be helped by its myriad medicinal forms. If we are truly concerned about a drug's effect on our teen's brain, then we should be just as circumspect in using FDA-approved pharmaceuticals that affect the developing brain. As I experienced in interacting with caretakers of sick teens, some disease symptoms are so severe that the number of pharmaceuticals needed reaches a point of diminishing—and tragic—returns.

Incurable

I never met Heather, but in the six months that I helped her mother treat her disease on a daily basis, I felt as though Heather were a close family friend. Heather, like her father, suffered from a torturous and ruthless genetic mutation called juvenile Huntington's disease (JHD). It is rare and it is incurable. Some say it is similar to having ALS, Parkinson's, and Alzheimer's all at once. Heather's father discovered he had Huntington's disease when symptoms developed in his forties. When Heather's mother Nancy came to me, he had been in a twenty-four-hour care facility for several years, leaving her alone with Heather, who was diagnosed with JHD at sixteen. To say that Nancy was at her wit's end was an understatement. Nancy's doctors fed dozens of pharmaceuticals to Heather to manage the convulsions and muscle spasms she experienced. She was on meds for infections, rashes, pain, and insomnia. Some of these prescriptions addressed the symptoms of her disease and some addressed the side effects of other medications. They didn't know where the JHD ended and the drug side effects began. Heather fell continually, she had intractable pain and itching, and she could barely hold down food. The drugs made her nauseous. Her life expectancy was only a few years, but her quality of life was almost nonexistent.

If ever there was a teenager who could benefit from the euphoric side effects of cannabis, it is one suffering from JHD or other terminal illnesses who has little hope for comfort. But euphoria was low on the list of Heather's needs. First, she needed to eat and sleep. She needed to reduce painful spasms, and she wanted pain relief. In creating formulations for Heather, I worked with her mom to ease into the products slowly. Using an infused oil that I created from my more sedative strains of cannabis, Nancy would put a drop or two on a piece of toast and observe the result with Heather after several hours. Despite THC's ability to have an immediate effect in terms of psychoactivity, pain, and appetite, the oils and cannabinoids can take longer to penetrate tissues. Each day, there would be a text exchange between Nancy and me as we tweaked the time of ingestion or changed titration over several hours or days. After assessing the results, I would advise her to take the oils at a later time of day if she was sluggish or to back off from the dose if it stimulated her and she had trouble sleeping. As I discovered with other patients, what Heather had in her stomach, the time of day she took her dose, what medium the cannabinoids were infused into, and her mindset all altered the response to the cannabis. As I helped guide Heather's use based on her day-to-day symptoms, the results began to be more positive. Soon, the rash medications decreased, then stopped. Powerful opioids Heather took for pain could be taken less frequently, and her sleep meds collected dust on her nightstand. Nancy was empowered and armed with daytime and nighttime tinctures, topicals, and healthy edibles that Heather liked to eat. Their relationship was better, and she concluded that both she and Heather were feeling more hopeful.

When law enforcement raided my home—taking my unique medicinal cannabis strains and dozens of tinctures, oils, and even CBD products—Heather no longer had access to the cannabis that managed her symptoms. Nancy promptly wrote a letter to the prosecutor to support my legal case. Sometimes a mother's words can more effectively explain how a medicine we dismiss as "weed" can alter the course of a life.

To Whom It May Concern:

I am writing this email on behalf of Ezra Parzybok. For those unaware, JHD is a neurodegenerative disease that robs one of the ability to walk, talk, eat, and do everything that one takes advantage of doing on a daily basis. After her diagnosis, my daughter declined at an alarming rate. Her neurologist prescribed medicine to help with neuropathy, restlessness, and seizures. My daughter had not been sleeping, had been losing weight, and had been downright uncomfortable and miserable. I was advised to see Ezra for a consultation, and, upon speaking with him, had realized that he had learned more about JHD in the day before I saw him, than many of her doctors have known since her being a patient of theirs. He suggested an oil to help with itching and restlessness, as well as one to help her sleep. I tried each. They did not help right away. However, upon using consistently, and consulting with Ezra, we came to a dosage that made a HUGE difference in my daughter's ability to live every day life. She was also doing much better with sleep. It was truly amazing. Her school tutors as well as her OT and PT's were amazed at the difference in her. It seemed too good to be true. It wasn't a miracle cure, but it did make a HUGE POSITIVE IMPACT on her daily life and well-being.

Fast forward to today. We can no longer receive treatment from Ezra. My daughter has been in the hospital since the end of July. She was hospitalized due to a rash that we could not get rid of, as well as skin ulcers and an unbearable itch. She had a yeast infection from an antibiotic given for the rash. She's not had the benefit of Ezra's oils, so she continues to fight with sleeping, in spite of the psychiatrist and neurologist prescribing different sleep medications. She continues to struggle with neuropathy and cannot sit down, So she lies on mats on the hospital floor. She's had two seizures since her admittance, in spite of the doctors trying to find the "right" anti-seizure medication. It has been a nightmare because the meds are coming with a whole new list of side effects. She has lost eight pounds because she has no appetite from all of the medications that she needs to be on for her list of issues.... JHD patients need between 5,000–6,000 calories per day so that they don't LOSE weight. She now weighs 80 lbs, and that is on a good day. This is such a rapid disease that I want to be able to love my baby for as long as I can.

In closing, I beg of you to allow Ezra to continue helping those who have truly benefited from his remedies. Clearly, there are bigger fish to catch. Please, please, do not convict Ezra.

Sincerely,
A Concerned Mother

Nancy's anonymous letter, and those of many patients, helped sway the prosecutor's case against me in my favor. I am forever indebted to them. But the leniency in my case did nothing for Nancy or Heather. I texted her about three weeks after I was raided. Heather and other clients who had been cut off from my services were weighing on my mind.

She responded later that day: "Ezra, Heather passed away Monday night. She is now resting and at peace. There are no words. No parent should ever have to endure such unbelievable heartache."

On the Spectrum

As Heather's case shows, many physical symptoms can be brought into check with the regulating effects of cannabinoids. Disorders of the mind are more challenging, as they can be frustratingly difficult to diagnose and treat. If a mildly autistic teenager has trouble getting out of bed in the morning, is it a symptom of his autism, or is he just being a teenager? Or perhaps it is merely a rebellious reaction to his disapproving mother, a type A morning person. A doctor who has spent a lifetime learning the intricacies of neurobiology and pharmacology may treat the behavior with a stimulant like Adderall (an amphetamine also known as "speed"). Or she may prescribe an antidepressant like Prozac to pull the child out of his doldrums. For many patients, regardless of the controversy of giving mind-altering drugs to teenagers, these drugs may just do the trick. For Eric, the sixteen-year-old autistic boy that was brought to me by his mother Krista, these drugs were anything but successful. According to Krista and him, when he took conventional drugs, his anxiety and depression were exacerbated and would spike erratically, yet his usual creativity and passion for games and puzzles dwindled.

A generation ago, Eric would be described as *idiosyncratic*. On the playground, he might have been referred to by the less erudite term "weirdo." But in an age of highly educated moms and the immense increase in autism diagnoses, Eric is a classic example of a kid "on the spectrum." Shy and lurching in his movements, with hesitation around new places or change in routine, Eric came to my door timidly. Wearing a white t-shirt and jeans, he clutched a heavily used water bottle that slung over his shoulder. It was one of those wide-mouth, hard plastic types, but it had been duct-taped, battered, and taped again. It was his security blanket and a visual representation of his obsessive-compulsive disorder (OCD). He never left home without it. Eric was the only child in a progressive, well-educated, and worldly family.

Krista had just dealt with the heart-wrenching stress of watching her child wean himself from selective serotonin reuptake inhibitors (SSRIS, a form of antidepressants) and other drugs. She just managed to wean Eric from them before he succumbed to his suicidal thoughts. (I didn't ask how far those thoughts took him, but his mother recounted it somberly.) Many studies have confirmed that SSRIS and antidepressants are about as effective as a placebo for adults.[8] Paradoxically, in children they've been linked to an increase in suicidal ideation.[9] SSRIS can lead to suicidal thoughts, violence, exacerbated symptoms, and other harmful side effects.[10] She was now at square one, and since the medical marijuana law passed, she thought she'd have Eric give cannabis a try. The legalities are somewhat tedious. In Massachusetts at the time, she could *procure* medical marijuana for Eric's ailments as long she filled out twice as much paperwork and saw twice as many doctors, all of whom were about as reticent about marijuana as they were cavalier about pharmaceuticals.

My first session with Eric and Krista consisted primarily of a debate between me and Eric about the morality of teenagers' using cannabis when it was a federally illegal drug. Why should an upstanding teenager do something that was illegal? He was smart—and cautious. I respected his trepidation, yet I had spent a decade responding to teenagers' skepticism about everything under the sun. I was unattached to his response, and I had all the time in the world to lay out the facts. First, I told him about some of the history of cannabis as a medication.

"Cannabis tinctures like mine were available in pharmacies all over the country for almost a hundred years. From 1850 to 1940, you could ask the pharmacist for something to help with a toothache, cramps, or in your case, calming your mind and helping you focus, and he might give you a small bottle of cannabis extract to try," I explained. I realized this didn't really address why it was illegal, so I paused and let him ask the question.

"Well then, why is it illegal now? Is it because it's addictive or because of how it makes you feel? That's what I'm worried about. I just don't want to get high. I don't want to feel that," he said.

"Honey, you don't have to get stoned. That's what I've been saying. You just take a little bit!" Said Krista, barely keeping her impatience at bay.

"Those are good questions, Eric. And you're smart to do research and ask as many questions as you can. It can be addictive when it causes a euphoric or 'high' side effect. It's not physically addictive like alcohol or opium, but you know what the hardest addiction is to kick?"

"No, what's that?" he asked.

"It's the one you have. For some, it's marijuana—usually the kind that's smoked. Cough syrup is a similar example. A small dose can help your cough. A large dose can get you high. You might focus better if cannabis is in your system, but ideally you won't feel the effects at all. As far as why it's illegal— that's a bigger discussion. Technically, if you have your medical marijuana card, it's not illegal. That's the point. But why it's illegal in general is more about politics than it is about the safety of the medicine. For example, the antidepressant you were on *is* legal but as you experienced—"

"I'm not taking those again," Eric interrupted, with a cold stare.

He left that session neutral on the subject and said he would "think about it." I was in no hurry to illegally provide cannabis to a sixteen-year-old, but I also empathized with his mother. She had watched him hit rock bottom with pharmaceuticals. He was an intelligent and gentle boy, and I loved the challenge. According to the law, I was dealing drugs to children in a school zone. But according to my thinking, as well as Krista's, we were puzzling out a way to help Eric progress in his life using a natural medicine.

There is a wide spectrum of altered consciousness when it comes to cannabis. Smoking, although effective for many, is akin to killing a cockroach with a sledgehammer when it comes to shifting the behavior of a reserved and docile autistic boy. If he decided to try cannabis at all, I would start him on a cold-processed glycerin tincture. I had been given some by a colleague several months back, and it stuck out in my mind as a possibility since everyone who had tried it noticed precisely no effect whatsoever. The process consists of putting some dried leaves or flowers into vegetable glycerin and letting it sit for several weeks. The glycerin slowly becomes infused with raw cannabinoids, and the result is a very light dose of primarily THCA. The "A" stands for THC's acidic form. It is the precursor molecule to THC and is basically nonpsychoactive. The body slowly breaks it down into THC, so one could theoretically get high with enough of it, but it would require downing a whole bottle of the stuff. Despite his mother's impatience with Eric, the last thing I wanted to do was give him a bad trip.

A couple of weeks later, Eric came to me again after having dedicated extensive Internet time to cannabis research. He had ultimately acclimated to the idea that cannabis in small doses was relatively harmless. He was still worried it was going to get him high, so I explained my dosing strategy.

"Generally, it takes a tincture or even an edible anywhere from twenty minutes to two hours to feel the effects. So the most conservative method of titrating is to take a small dose early in the day and then assess its effects over twenty-four hours. Then, the following day, you can go up if needed. You can start with as little as one drop." I was confident he could take a swig out of the bottle and not have an adverse reaction, but you never know. "Here, I'll take a drop right now on my finger like so." I unscrewed the dropper bottle, eased out a drop, and licked my finger.

"I would be surprised if you felt anything with such a small dose, but I suppose it's conceivable." I smacked my lips innocently to downplay the images he might have in his head from the Internet and handed the tincture to his mom. She did the same. After explaining in depth how he should use it and what he should expect to feel—a reduction of symptoms versus an increase in sensation—I told him to think it over and walked them both to the door.

"Eric, your water bottle. Geez, don't forget that!" said Krista as she retrieved it from the couch. She looked at me in exasperation, while Eric wandered distractedly down the front steps. She stopped before leaving and turned to me. "You know, I'm kinda feeling that drop. Is that possible? It feels nice, actually. Maybe I should be the one getting a medical marijuana card!"

"You're feeling that one drop? It's surprising, but not impossible. It's actually helpful that you tried it. It will help for you to have a sense of its potency."

Several weeks later, Krista reported that about ten drops of glycerin seemed to take the edge off Eric's anxiety, although he didn't notice any physical effects from it. He had an easier time focusing in the morning, was more resilient to stress, and was better able to cope with the schedule at his school.

Krista ordered one last bottle of glycerin tincture for Eric a few hours before I was raided. When the marijuana dispensary opened in our area (six days later), they didn't have cold-processed glycerin tincture. Luckily, I was able to teach Krista to make it herself. She would buy cannabis flower buds from the dispensary that are typically used for smoking and cook them on low heat into glycerin. A year later, she wrote to tell me that Eric was thriving at his new school. She proudly shared that he had been invited to give his class graduation speech. It was received with much fanfare.

Violence to Self and Others

Another parent of an autistic child came to me for advice on her son, Corey, who was a nonverbal, severely autistic young man with anxiety and violent tendencies. Working with a patient like Corey was controversial because he was not able to verbalize what his needs were or what his response was to medications. His behavior could be observed only by those closest to him. Corey, like Eric, had been on a wide array of FDA-approved pharmaceuticals most of his life. Benzodiazapines, SSRIs, and other antipsychotic drugs filled his medicine cabinet. They had tried them all. But sadly, some conventional drugs can cause the same symptoms they are intended to address. Although the data are controversial, there is evidence to suggest that for some, antidepressants alone are thought to be responsible for violence, suicide, mania, and other forms of psychotic and bizarre behavior.[11] The suicidal ideation study cited found that "young adults between the ages of 15–24, were nearly fifty percent more likely to be convicted of a homicide, assault, robbery, arson, kidnapping, sexual offense and other violent crime when on the antidepressant than when they weren't taking the psychiatric drug."[12]

It seems counterintuitive that some drugs would cause the opposite effect of what they're prescribed for, but it may be due in part to the fact that some drugs can have what's called biphasic, bidirectional, or paradoxical effects. Some medications such as the class of drugs known as benzodiazapenes, which are often used to treat mood disorders,[13] have been shown to exacerbate symptoms in some patients.[14] Biphasic psychiatric drugs are problematic, to say the least. For one thing, psychiatric drugs are addressing the gray area of consciousness between sanity and insanity. This is difficult to do objectively. Many clients have come to me traumatized by the doctors, family members, and drugs that sought to address their psychosis effectively. They ended up feeling worse on the drugs and turned to cannabis because it helped where the others could not. Many are helped by the drugs, but as some long-term studies show, antipsychotic drugs don't ultimately help people reduce psychosis. For example, one study showed twice the recovery rate in patients who reduced or discontinued their drugs as those who managed their symptoms with antipsychotic drugs.[15] Another separate study concluded, "[Over twenty years, patients] not prescribed antipsychotics showed significantly less psychotic activity than those prescribed antipsychotics." Worse, some drugs might actually exacerbate psychosis when patients do discontinue use. Yet another study found that "psychosis may be a feature of drug withdrawal rather than the re-emergence of an underlying illness, at least in some patients."[16] I empathize with the patients and parents who have to decide whether to use antipsychotic medication. But if cannabis was part of a psychiatrist's prescriptive repertoire, perhaps it could be an option for some patients where other drugs had failed.

Of course, conventional drugs are helpful for many people, and cannabis is not a silver bullet. Cannabinoids have also shown biphasic properties in animal studies.[17] In humans, the number-one reported reason for using cannabis is for its relaxing and tension-relieving effects. And the number-one reported cause for ending cannabis use is because of its anxiety and panic-inducing effects.[18] I have noticed in clients that the effects of cannabis over time can also be biphasic. Where a remedy might be effective for sleep and anxiety relief for six months, it then begins to stop working and seems to cause insomnia and anxiety. My hypothesis is that the cannabinoids are regulating the body, but if the underlying symptoms are not addressed on a fundamental level, then the cannabinoids are ultimately not effective at blocking the message the body is sending. They regulate cell behavior as well as organism behavior. A patient's lifestyle or deeper symptoms could be lurking under the surface of the drug's effect, only to rear up later if not addressed.

Despite cannabinoids' potential for being biphasic, one benefit is that a patient can feel the effects somewhat rapidly. Corey needed something to help him unwind from his violent state and sleep through his nightmares. It also had to be something that his mother could readily observe as being effective. I suggested a slow-cooked, cannabis-infused olive oil made with a cured variety of indica (sedative) cannabis that she put into his food. I chose strains I knew to generally be relaxing because I had tried them myself or collected detailed reports from other clients based on their symptoms. Because I was the grower, I could observe the physiological structure of the plant as well, which helped me determine its effect. Cooking the oils for a long period of time—often for several days—diminished the psychoactivity of the THC.

The results for Corey were almost immediate. He started sleeping better and having fewer nightmares. His daytime activity was more balanced due to better sleep, and his violent outbursts dropped significantly. With as small a dose as a few drops of the sedative oil (approximately 2 mg of THC) stirred into his yogurt, Corey wasn't stoned, but his behavior change was noticed by his family and health aides. This is a scenario where keeping the child safe and alive is the priority. His mother wasn't worried about getting him into college. That was not an option. Any arguments about lost IQ or lack of motivation were useless for Corey's mom. Her top priority was preventing him from doing harm to himself or others. In comparison with the pharmaceuticals that elicit the opposite of their intended effect, for Corey's mom, using cannabis was not a difficult choice.

The Teen Brain Debate

The habitual pattern of thought stands in the way of other impressions.
Yoga Sutra Patanjali 1:50

For teens like Heather, Corey, and the circumspect Eric, choosing cannabis as medicine is less controversial. Using my simple approach of assessing what is available and comparing the prescription drugs side by side with properly formulated and dosed cannabis remedies, certainly a parent can see the benefits of treating cannabis as just another pharmaceutical option. But the pervasive debate surrounding cannabis and teens is not whether it should be a medicine for acutely ill children. I hope doctors and law enforcement have the sense to recognize that a parent like Nancy is merely asking for relief as she watches her only child die of a terminal disease.

But most parents are not dealing with terminally ill teenagers. Some teens' excessive smoking and arguments of "it's my medicine!" are driving many parents to drink, as it were. Parents have a right to be worried. The scientific debate on whether cannabis is permanently damaging a teen's developing brain is still unsettled as I write this. In 2012, a study concluded that "persistent cannabis users show neurological decline from childhood to midlife."[19]

This was based on a famous, long-term review of a cohort from Dunedin, New Zealand. It followed approximately one thousand kids into adulthood. Adjusting for many variables in the cohort, such as alcohol and tobacco use, the study ultimately based its findings on roughly sixty people. It made headlines worldwide and was a home run for the DEA.

In 2016, I attended a marijuana lecture entitled "Marijuana: What We Know, What We Don't Know" by a Harvard neuroscientist. Referencing the Dunedin study, she proceeded to detail all of the correlated harms of cannabis to a packed lecture hall at a prestigious college. Claiming no bias when the audience took her to task for her one-sidedness and lack of distinction between correlation and causation, she neglected to cite a 2014 study I found that came to the opposite conclusion about the effect of cannabis on youth. Published by the same *Proceedings of the National Academy of Sciences,* it also followed hundreds of children—this time twins—into adulthood. It concluded that "marijuana-using twins failed to show significantly greater IQ decline relative to their abstinent siblings."[20]

We assume that science is free from judgment and is purely data driven, but cannabis is elusive and research can be fraught with agendas. Scientists are not robots. They have opinions that are affected by stereotypes as well. Therefore, it is difficult to separate their assumptions about the plant from the data they collect. For example, the researcher who gave the lecture on cannabis was one of the lead Harvard neuroscientists on yet another study of cannabis effect on the brain. The Harvard study made headlines and was again a feather in the cap of the DEA stance on cannabis. Its title says it all: "Cannabis Use is Quantitatively Associated with [Brain] Abnormalities in Young Adult Recreational Users."[21] For millions of parents and health professionals who came across news referencing the study (with pictures of youths smoking joints, no doubt), the debate was settled. Pot is bad for teens and we should continue to arrest them for its use.

Other scientific studies have been performed in an attempt to replicate the results of the Harvard study, but they were not successful. One concludes via its title that "Daily Marijuana Use Is Not Associated with Brain Abnormalities in Adolescents or Adults."[22] Another study on the effects of cannabis on executive function further contradicts the cultural perception of marijuana's brain frying effects. Although the data are based on adult medical marijuana

(MMJ) patients, it concluded that "in general, MMJ patients experienced some improvement on measures of executive functioning, mostly reflected as increased speed in completing tasks without a loss of accuracy. Patients also reported a notable decrease in their use of conventional pharmaceutical agents from baseline, with opiate use declining more than forty-two percent."[23]

The results of these studies are precisely the opposite of the Harvard study. It seems science can find evidence on both sides of the argument. If you're a concerned parent of a teenager, by now you're probably more confused by the science than ever. Regardless of the complexity of determining the truth about cannabis use, the studies point to a more nuanced approach to how we might use and experience cannabis. It requires one to take a step back from the science and instead acknowledge that there may be some commonsense truth to both sides of the argument. For its conclusion may have little to do with what science can pin down and much more to do with culture, language, and, ultimately, how we parent.

Since cannabis is typically consumed in whole plant form and not as a processed, singular molecule, it is difficult to know if the pot one person smokes is making him dull witted, whereas the pot someone else smokes is making her ace a test. I have seen evidence of both. If researchers follow a bunch of teenagers around who smoke random pot smuggled from Mexico that is laced with banned pesticides like DDT, then this marijuana might be damaging the teens' brains. Even in the purest organic cannabis, there are more than four hundred distinct chemical compounds, and over sixty of them are active cannabinoids.[24] Cannabis that has ripened on the plant longer than average is generally considered to be more sedative or "stoney." Its cannabinoid profile can be different from a less ripe plant. A strain that one person grows lovingly in an organic soil mixture may produce a flower that allows a user to reduce debilitating ADD symptoms and focus on the work at hand. Another user of this same flower may instead focus on his shoelace for fifteen minutes, causing him to be late to gym class. It is my opinion that the scientific debate about both the harms of cannabis and its quantifiable medical efficacy will carry on for years to come. California has had legal medical marijuana for over twenty years, yet still there is no standardized dosing or list of strains that correspond consistently to specific ailments. California has many recreational users, but it also has many die-hard medical researchers who are trying to puzzle out this problem. I spoke to a chemist at a well-known cannabis testing laboratory in California who told me a single plant can be analyzed by two different labs and still have a 20 percent variance in terms of cannabinoid potency.[25] We can try to jam the square peg of cannabinoids into the round hole of precision medicine all we want. Rarely does the peg fit.

Psychological trauma is an ailment that points to some of the beneficial as well as harmful effects of cannabis on the teen brain. Trauma itself can have a lasting impact on the brain, leading to depression, anxiety, and symptoms of PTSD.[26] Many antidepressants prescribed to relieve these symptoms can take six weeks to have any effect on the body, and rarely are their side effects "euphoric."

A colleague of mine lost his father during his sophomore year at a boarding school. Although this was over forty years ago, pot was as readily available to him as it is today. After class, feeling numb from the loss and isolated from his peers, he would roll a joint and smoke it in the basement of his dormitory. Although he doesn't use cannabis now, he has always been grateful that cannabis helped him through that tough time. "It basically got me through my sophomore year of high school," he told me. He never became addicted, and it didn't affect his studies. He was appropriately self-medicating. He managed to eat, bathe, and study for his classes. His after-school joint eased the stress of keeping up appearances throughout the day and helped balance his nervous system for the following day.

When parents of teens come to me now to ask my advice about the subtleties of use versus abuse, I maintain a conservative stance. The brain is still developing, and they should be aware that heavy cannabis use, even though it may not be damaging the brain, can be debilitating. If the teen is recovering from a trauma in his life, then using the drug may not be holding him back. If it's helping him forget the trauma and move on with his studies, then it would be difficult to convince him that it's "damaging," even if it may be affecting his memory adversely. Although a comprehensive 2013 study found that short-term memory can be negatively affected by cannabis use,[27] the correlation between the two is not always one-to-one. According to the study, "chronic exposure of cannabinoid drugs may result in the development of tolerance [in the brain] to the adverse effects of THC." Also, "THC acutely decreased performance in the [executive functioning] in occasional users [but] no such performance deficits were reported in heavy smokers following administration of the same dose." In essence, we seem to know that marijuana affects memory—and most users will tell you that they are more forgetful while on the drug—but it's difficult to nail down the exact effect across the board for all users. Although the science is hard to pin down, education and communication, not criminalization, is a better approach.

If a teen finds that it is a more effective medication than pharmaceuticals, I would still recommend that the cannabis remedy have CBD as well as THC to reduce psychoactivity yet still soften the traumatic memories. Changing dosing to a more appropriate microdose during the day and working with an informed mental health professional for trauma or PTSD support could shift use from an essentially recreational relationship with the drug to a medicinal one. Today, with strains having more concentrated amounts of THC, smoking a blunt or a joint usually provides far more cannabinoids to the user than what's needed. The goal should be to reduce the stress and then reduce the medication. After a few months, weaning the user off THC and increasing CBD-dominant remedies would be an ideal choice. As long as the teen is moving forward in his or her studies and evolving emotionally, memory intact, a proper dose of cannabinoids could be an acceptable option to address the trauma.

If depression and cannabis consumption persists, then it's an issue that needs to be addressed. The goal of my practice is to reduce my patients' symptoms, reduce harmful medication, and increase quality of life. Teenagers and anyone working through grief should seek help from a professional, but if the conventional medical approach to these ailments is brain-altering drugs that take six weeks to be as effective as a placebo, then cannabis should be considered an option.

A high school kid medicating with cannabis is controversial because teens already exist in a culture immersed in the recreational use of cannabis. Our intuition tells us that we don't want kids having more excuses to use cannabis. (For a soldier, reporter, or aid worker returning from a war zone or an adult with a history of trauma, a proper dose of cannabis that eases PTSD-like symptoms is a no-brainer.) But two studies on cannabinoids may prove the benefits in treating injuries of the brain at all ages. A study on humans suffering with traumatic brain injury (TBI) found that those who had the cannabinoid THC in their system had a significantly lower mortality rate than those who had no THC.[28] Cannabinoids have also been shown to promote neurogenesis, or the creation of new brain cells, in adult mice. In order to test a synthetic cannabinoid drug intended for use in brain trauma, mice were given a dose of a cannabinoid after a traumatic brain injury. The results were promising. Owing to the creation and protection of the brain cells, "although given at 7 days post injury, these effects [were] associated with significant neuroprotective effects, leading to an improvement in neurobehavioral functions."[29] Furthermore, in a separate study it is suggested that this positive effect on the brain helps promote the mood-balancing effects of cannabinoids observed in mice. The finding that mice have a decrease in anxiety and depressive symptoms leads to the conclusion that cannabinoid-promoted neurogenesis may contribute to anxiolytic and antidepressive effects.[30] Many football players in the National Football League are advocating for the legal use of the drug to reduce TBI and chronic traumatic encephalopathy, a condition experienced by boxers, football players, and other athletes who have continual impacts to the brain. If your teenager plays football, a few puffs with friends after practice may be having a net protective effect.

The brain is plastic in nature, and experiences (whether trauma induced or conditioned by our lifestyle) can alter neuronal patterns in the brain.[31] So patterned responses, and therefore the synapses that recreate these patterns, are built and destroyed based on our thoughts. The neuroscientists Richard Semon and Donald Hebb studied how cells assemble themselves in patterns and create connections. Their work led to the phrase "the cells that fire together wire together."[32] The idea is that as synapses form, the ones that are continually activated become stronger and more active. If the cannabis user is not wiring productive synapses by enacting healthy activity and healthy thoughts, could the cannabis be reinforcing the synapses patterned to perpetuate the unhealthy state?

For example, if you *think* a bomb is going off every time you hear a door slam, then synapses build that patterned response in your brain. If instead you can slow down that fight-or-flight memory with cannabis—as well as promote new neurons—and then train your mind to *think* of the banal circumstances of the noise, then the idea is that the PTSD-associated pattern of synapses will wither and the new pattern will emerge. Thus, your brain on cannabis is not an egg frying in a skillet. It may be more like a choose-your-own-adventure.

If we are raising generally well-rounded teenagers who are not fighting terminal illness, trauma, grief, or mood disorders, we might find that occasional cannabis use can enhance their curiosity and deep thinking. Teenagers are transitioning from childhood to adulthood. They are working hard to catch the bus, do their homework, and avoid the chores their parents put upon them. When 4:20 p.m.—the now infamous numeric code for all things cannabis—arrives after school, pot can provide a way to escape the busy world and embrace the comforting and often fascinating cell behavior that is occurring naturally inside their bodies. Cannabinoids within our body—and the bodies of fish, emus, and elephants—are first and foremost regulators of cell behavior. Regardless of the plant, our internal cannabinoids are perpetually seeking to balance the behavior of the nervous system and the immune system. We all want balance in our lives, and it makes perfect sense that many teenagers (and adults) would gravitate toward a sensation that makes them feel at ease and that connects them with nature, as some describe. It gives their whirring mind a rest. Is this a bona fide antidepressant? For some, yes.

What we do know about the young brain is that it is still developing well into adulthood. Some might argue that complete abstinence from marijuana until one's late twenties is the safest way to avoid potential harm to the brain. But because the science is not settled, it's possible that moderate marijuana use at the time of life when young, productive adults are differentiating from their parents and are exploring new ideas and delving deeper into the nature of their own minds is actually beneficial to the brain. Regardless of the measurable effects on the brain, millions of teens will experiment with cannabis anyway. If we as a culture can provide space in the home to talk about healthy and appropriate cannabis use, then I believe the teen brain will benefit.

It is when life goes out of balance and remains so that the harms of cannabis can manifest. Repeated traumas in childhood—death in the family, social isolation, or even the added stress of poverty—can make the desire to seek out and abuse cannabis more appealing. Teens find that cannabis provides a buffer from these chronic stresses. They then become addicted to this buffer, fearful of the inner work required to grow, change, and heal. The world feels safer behind it. In my opinion, smoking a puff or two after class to deal with the grief of a lost parent is a viable medicinal response to an ailment. A weekly session with a therapist in whom the student can confide would compound and sustain the medicinal benefits. But if the daily joint turns into a twenty-four-hour high six months later and worsening grades, then that medication is no longer increasing quality of life. The brain may be experiencing harm. This can be described as "marijuana use disorder," and it affects about 1.5 percent of adults,[33] compared with 7 percent of adults who have "alcohol use disorder."[34] Parents need to have an open dialogue, and school administrators need a nuanced view of how cannabis is used by their students. To expel a student in this scenario might send him careening off balance in his life, increasing the desire to escape through cannabis or harder drugs.

The primary harm of cannabis, as with any vice from video games to sex to sugar, is abuse and addiction. We know that automobiles are dangerous to teenagers and the community members subjected to their dangerous driving, but that is why we have driving school and licenses and rules and regulations. Despite the danger of cars, they, like cannabis, can take teens to beautiful places. Still, we take our teenagers to an empty parking lot and teach them to drive. We don't make automobiles illegal. We make them safer and we make the laws take into account the causal evidence. Society has systems in place for dangerous things teenagers encounter. We have no reasonable system in place to address teenagers who smoke pot. Alarmist, antidrug pamphlets have been disseminated for generations. Teens will smoke it whether the science is definitive or not.

The legislatures may over- or undercorrect in creating marijuana laws, but without proper guidance from authorities, parents have to seek factual information and make decisions based on what is best for their family. Their relationship with and parenting of their teen is a subjective experience, not an objective one defined entirely by science. At a lecture I gave on cannabis, a concerned mom made the comment that she supported medical cannabis, but this did not help her with her pot-smoking teenage son.

"For God sakes," she said, "of course sick people should be allowed to try medical marijuana. But my seventeen-year-old is healthy and this is his brain we're talking about! I actually saw a text on his phone that said, '*Dude it's the last day of summer. Let's get as high as possible!!!*' I just don't know what to do! He is going to college next fall!" She placed her head in her hands in despair.

Because the science in this area is contradictory, I offered an analogy to help understand the harms of cannabis: think of growing up as a series of plateaus, I told her. As you mature, you reach a new plateau. The goal is always to reach the next plateau, but obstacles may arise, such as the loss of a family member, or something subtle like social isolation, or lack of purpose during summer months. A teen can become stuck in a rut, unable to evolve to the next plateau. Cannabis can break the user out of the rut and allow a creative leap to the next plateau. I've seen it happen in my adult patients, and I've heard stories of cannabis having this effect on people in their youth. I had a depressed client who had pursued nature photography at one time but hadn't picked up a camera for months, until she smoked a little cannabis to alleviate the pain from a lower leg amputation. Hours after smoking for the first time, she was walking in the woods, taking nature photos, and feeling hope again. She'd forgotten her creative block and her leg pain for a spell. Her mind was experiencing positive thoughts and new synaptic patterns. The euphoria experienced, as cannabis disperses attachments and releases dopamine, can be liberating. It opens people up to possibility and positivity.

"I have read every study on teen cannabis use and the developing brain," I told her. "Going by your demographic and the fact that he is a good student, it's unlikely your seventeen-year-old son is permanently damaging his brain." Her body relaxed—she was clearly relieved. "But it may be driving a wedge between the two of you. If you cannot connect with your son, or if the only argument you have is that it is damaging his brain, he may rebel further. He may use cannabis to buffer himself from the authority figures in his life, cutting off access to the community that supports him. This can be damaging."

If the teenager reaches for weed every time he struggles on the current plateau, the cannabis can therefore *become* the rut. Synapses wired to unhealthy activity fire as cannabis is consumed, releasing just enough endorphins to reinforce the bad habit. But the synapses associated with these feelings of depression, social anxiety, ennui, and so on may be getting stronger and stronger, especially given the evidence that cannabinoids are a neuroprotective. If this rut is felt by the user or observed by their supportive family and friends, then he or she must consider eliminating cannabis from the equation to allow the next plateau to be reached. Positive thoughts, actions, and healthy synapses need to form independently.

Once the person has arrived atop the next plateau of life unimpeded, cannabis can again help strengthen healthy synapses and guide one to the next level. Or, it can cause another rut. Some people get high every day and maintain a four-point grade average or put in sixty hours a week at the law firm. Many daily smokers are evolving as productive citizens. Teens may be more at risk, not for the purported measurable effects of cannabis on the brain, but for the way they use it to address or escape from the emotional struggles they have in school with socializing, finding identity, and progressing in their emotional development as individuals. If they are evolving socially and emotionally, then the cannabis they use is probably not impeding development, but only the individuals and those close to them can judge if they're evolving to the next plateau. If we are to settle the teen brain debate scientifically, then the important aspects that frame teenage experience, as well as sedative or stimulating strains, cure time, and processing methods, have to be taken into account to gain accurate information.

I am aware that a metaphor for brain development such as *plateau* or *rut* is not scientific language. But it is parental language. We must validate the pot use for its diverse positive effects, and we must hold the teen and ourselves to high standards, as it were. If a teen has a diagnosable disease, it makes the cannabis easier to "prescribe." But if the teen is healthy, how do you know if her cannabis use is appropriate? The parent can perform a simple experiment: request that the teen take a break from cannabis. Start with a forty-eight-hour break. This is often enough time to reset the cannabinoid receptors in the body. Tolerance decreases, and the user needs less THC to get the desired results. If a break is impossible, then abuse (or a diagnosable ailment) may be evident. The teen may be addicted to the illusion of progression that cannabis has created. Instead, cannabis is holding her back, and there may be a developmental plateau that is not being reached. If the teen can take a break for a week—or better, a month—then her use is probably safe. Better still, the parents can sit down with the teen and propose that the whole family take a break from a vice they feel entitled to. Parents will not convince a teen to stop smoking pot if they can't stop drinking wine every night with dinner. My family takes two weeks out of the year, one in fall and one in spring, to stop sugar, alcohol, cannabis, caffeine, meat, dairy, and other mood-enhancing substances that require moderation. I am not perfect, but I want my kids to know that I take my psychological and emotional development seriously. I strive to model it for them.

A parent I know who is a health professional encountered a common cannabis issue when his fourteen-year-old daughter shared that she had been offered cannabis at a party. The conversation came up as I had expressed to him that I hoped my children would avoid cannabis until their late twenties. He and his wife laughed. "Good luck with that!" they said and educated me on the realities of raising a teen.

Their daughter didn't know the older boy who offered the marijuana, and she ultimately declined his offer, but she brought the story back to her father because he hadn't kept his cannabis use secret. Being aware of the science, as well as the reality of raising a teenager, he had introduced his daughter to the subject gradually over the years. As he knew might happen, the pressure of her peers was beginning to exert itself. She was curious to know what it felt like to smoke marijuana. Since she was being solicited by unknown young men in the community to try it, her father had to take manners into his own hands.

"In that moment I had to decide what was more appropriate: Do I let random men lure my daughter into smoking pot with them or should I be the one to introduce it to her? How can I know she is safe when she tries it for the first time?" It is a difficult question to answer. I do not yet have teenagers living under my roof, so I do not claim to know the right answer. But I would have to agree with him that teenagers introducing teenagers to cannabis does not seem safer than letting a concerned parent doing so. It has been over a year since he chose the "safer" route. They are able to monitor her use because she feels safe sharing it with them. They remain connected on the subject and will be there if overuse becomes a problem.

The conversation about cannabis and taking a break from a vice is not easy, because it requires deeper thinking about one's life goals and life purpose. The talk about developmental plateaus becomes a spiritual conversation. It requires adult thinking and emotional intelligence. If the teen (or parent, for that matter) cannot understand the analogy, cannot articulate or meet her goals for the near future, or self-reflect on spiritual, emotional, and mental development, then in my eyes, she has lost the debate. It is time to seek help from a professional whom the teen and parent can trust. Psychiatrists who equate cannabis use with narcotic addiction may be missing the subtleties of the plant and the science of the endocannabinoid system. Perhaps it's a family friend or local cannabis consultant who can guide the teen toward taking a break. The goal should be less medication, fewer symptoms, and increased quality of life.

Regardless of the data on the subject, the teen brain and the curative or harmful aspects of cannabis may remain subjective. Cannabis can cure some people of disorders related to the brain, but like many pharmaceuticals, it may exacerbate those disorders, too.

It can be difficult to know if cannabis is harming the person who won't get a job and move out of his parents' basement. If he has a mental disorder, assessing the positive or negative effect of the chronic cannabis use can be more difficult. Does he need tough love, or would he be suicidal and violent on other forms of medication, or no cannabis at all? When arguments of health become subjective, we need a way to know objectively whether a person can be a productive member of society. How much of his disease actually is a result of an ailing mind? What symptoms are brought up to the doctor in the hope that the physician will just fix it for him with a magic pill? Because we have insurance companies deciding what they'll pay for, doctors prescribing the medications given to them by for-profit pharmaceutical companies, and individuals carrying their own baggage into doctor's visits, we often don't know how to unravel fact from fiction in treating disease. Doctors can't force patients to eat healthily, just as patients can't force insurance companies to pay for their yoga classes, even though both things can encourage health. We have to decide whether our health is in the hands of the system or whether it is in our hands—or both.

Some patients come to me for information about using cannabis for a symptom like pain and give me a detailed spreadsheet of all the medications they take for various ailments. One such example of a daily medication list from a middle-aged woman dealing primarily with debilitating nerve pain is illustrated in Table 1.

I put a check mark next to all of the symptoms that could potentially be addressed by a properly formulated cannabinoid remedy. If she already took over twenty medications on a daily basis and neither she nor her doctors thought this was a problem, then it was unlikely cannabis alone was going to address her symptoms. It was probably going to be just another medication on her list. It is at this point that patients have to think deeply about how much they believe in their body's miraculous ability to thrive and heal and overcome symptoms of disease. Although we don't quite know how or why it all happens, we are organisms of trillions of cells striving to live and carry on despite what nature, genetics, and our lifestyle throws at us. Are our individual personalities driving our ailments when we are sick, or is it the vessel that carries us—our body—that breaks down or gets damaged? Ailments of the mind are more complex, but how many of the symptoms in the list in Table 1 are physical and how many are perpetuated by a mental response? How many of the symptoms are side effects of the other medications? There are millions of people living this way. The modern medical system is a miracle of scientific achievement, but all the pills in the world cannot address the problem of personal responsibility for one's health. As a cannabis consultant and health practitioner, I am aware of the gray area between helping and hindering. Some cannabis users are perpetuating their ailments, and some doctors are perpetuating disease and discomfort by prescribing more pills.

My client James was an interesting case illuminating this gray area. He had no such list of medications and was never diagnosed with a mental disorder, but his social anxiety and agoraphobia were extreme. After going through a difficult breakup and dropping out of college with a large amount of debt, he found himself living back at home with his parents, unsure what to do with his life. He had been anxious since high school, where his timid and creative personality was beaten down repeatedly by a barrage of insults from more aggressive students. If he felt brave enough to say something in class, he was chastised. His older brothers were type A and had little empathy for his shy and nervous demeanor. When he attended college, he pursued political science, because the injustices of the world tortured him and he was

TABLE 1 *The gray area of help versus harm*

NAME	DOSE	COUNT	INSTRUCTIONS	PRESCRIBED FOR
Buspirone HCL	5mg	Take 1	3x a day	Depression
Dronabinol	5mg	Take 1-5	Up to 3x daily as needed	Nausea and Vomiting
Humulin (insulin)	2 Units	Per sliding scale	350-400 take 6 units	High Blood Sugar. *Call Dr. If blood sugar over 400
Lantus (insulin long-acting	22 Units	1 Injection	At bedtime	Long-Acting Insulin
Lipitor	80mg	Take 1	Morning	Cholesterol
Lisinopril	20mg	Take 1	Morning	High Blood Pressure
Meclizine	25mg	Take 1-2	As needed	Dizziness, Nausea
Metformin HCL	500mg	Take 2 Take 1	Morning Before Dinner	Diabetes
Metoprolol Succ ER	50mg	Take 1	Bedtime	Hypertension
Morphine ER	60mg	Take 1	Bedtime	Pain
Oxazepam	10mg	Take 1-2 Take 1-5	Up to 3x daily Bedtime	Muscle Spasms Sleep
Ranitidine	300mg	Take 1	3x Daily	Acid Reflux
Singulair SOD	10mg	Take 1	Bedtime	Breathing
Effexor	225mg	Take 1	Morning	Depression
Zofran	8mg	Take 2	Morning	Nausea Vomiting
Flo-nase	50mcg	1 Spray	Each Nostril	Sinitus/Allergies
Pro-Air	90mcg	2 puffs	As needed every 4 hours	Wheezing
Symbicort		1 puff	2x daily	Chronic Bronchitis
Clobetasol	.05%	Small dab	2x daily	Psoriasis
Emla Cream	30gm	Every 12 hours	As needed	Extreme Pain
Lidocaine Patch	5%	Every 12 hours	As needed	Extreme Pain
PBK Cream	60ml	Apply 1-2 cc to painful area	As needed	Extreme Pain
Tolnaflate Powder	1%	1-2 times daily	To affected area	Yeast skin infection

determined to help make it a better place. But when he followed his friends to political rallies and protests, his social anxiety incapacitated him. He had tried antidepressants and antianxiety drugs, but either he had experienced difficult side effects, such as insomnia and increased suicidal thoughts, or the drugs did little to aid him.

When he smoked pot for the first time in college, he immediately wondered if the trajectory of his life would have been different if he'd discovered it sooner. On cannabis, he felt a buffer from fear, his shyness faded, and his central nervous system ratcheted down its fight-or- flight response by several notches. Tragically, his therapist had passed away a year before he came to me, and he had not found anyone to talk to who could understand his cannabis usage or help peel back the layers of fear and anxiety. His mother, Cathy, called me to find out whether his cannabis intake could be tweaked in order to help him move forward in his life. I gave him the usual information about using daytime strains for the day and nighttime strains at night and recommended he consider alternative forms such as CBD and ingestible oils, which could mitigate his anxiety more effectively than smoking. I didn't hear back until Cathy called me more than a year later out of desperation. He had been living in their basement for nineteen months, stuck in a holding pattern of self-loathing, indecision, and self-medicating with marijuana.

"I just don't know what to do with him. He's such a talented kid. And smart. But now all he does is smoke pot all day. I know it helps him, because I can see the difference if he doesn't, but he's just stuck. He won't look for a job, he doesn't come up when people come over, and he sure won't talk to me. After his therapist died he said you're the only one he felt a connection with. Can you help?"

I was surprised to get the call, but I knew few therapists would have a nuanced approach to his self-medicating, so I began seeing him regularly. James and I began our weekly sessions much as a therapist and client would. He would sit in my office and fidget, while I asked him questions about his symptoms, how he used cannabis, and what he might do to break out of his rut and progress in his life. My goal was still conservative. I believed that the cannabis did mitigate his worst symptoms of panic and anxiety, but I wanted him to work up to a forty-eight-hour break, in order to reset his THC tolerance. I suggested he start adding CBD to his regimen and explained my theory that the high-THC cannabis, although beneficial for some symptoms, might be preventing his mind from breaking out of its rut. It might have been exacerbating his anxiety.

The interesting thing about James was that he was not a typical pothead. He didn't just wake up and take bong hits, then proceed to while away his day in a stupor. He exercised regularly, played classical piano, read philosophical texts extensively, and longed to take a tolerance break so that he could reset his cannabinoid receptors. He rarely felt high anymore and no longer attained the peaceful, inspiring highs he had experienced in college. Now he was just medicating to get through his day.

I felt James was capable of breaking out of his rut if he could reset his tolerance, take a substantial break, and move to a new plateau of development. Then he could pursue cannabis again for symptom relief or recreation, once he'd exited the vicious cycle he was manifesting. I was also torn about my prognosis. If the medical cannabis he was taking was working to keep his worst ailments at bay, then why should he go off the medication? The idea is not foreign to many people who hate the pills they take. I had seen patients who had taken an effective drug but still wanted to wean themselves from it because they had a feeling that it was hurting their liver, or could lead to other symptoms. It can be demoralizing to be dependent on a drug, whatever its effect.

In James's case, I felt that the potential side effect of not progressing in his life was too severe. If my hypothesis was correct, James was stuck in a cannabis catch-22. The drug was the most effective medication for reducing symptoms of anxiety, but it was also perpetuating his anxiety and self-loathing. He was living as a stereotype of a pothead in his parents' basement. He was ashamed of his status, ashamed of his debt, and had no career to help him escape. I assumed that many people like James medicated with other, stronger prescription drugs and still didn't progress in their lives. They managed their symptoms, but the side effects of the drug, their lifestyle, or their ailments were still too severe to allow them go get a job and move on with their development. I believed James was stable and healthy enough to break the cycle if he could lift the needle on the broken record of marijuana consumption.

We talked at length about his daily routine and his process of medicating. He would wake up at about eight in the morning, shower, and eat breakfast.

At about ten, he would go for a jog or head to the gym for a workout (as long as he could interact with people as little as possible). At about midafternoon his anxious thoughts would intrude, and he was no longer able to keep his guilt, shame, fear, and panic at bay. The world was in turmoil, and he was a loser, living at his parent's house in a small, conservative town. He was lonely. He was penniless. Hives would even break out across his neck and face. He would shut down, his parents unable to reach him. His despondency was palpable. And then, regretfully, he'd smoke pot. In the first hour or two, the positive effects always outweighed the negative. His mind was at ease, the hives subsided, and he could go back to playing Chopin on the grand piano in his basement. I trusted that he wanted to stop, and I also believed that the cannabis truly helped him manage his mental anguish. But the longest James was able to abstain from cannabis was about eighteen hours. Eventually, he stopped coming for our "therapy" sessions. He felt guilty that his mom had to drive him (his panic attacks made driving dangerous), and his agoraphobia worsened. His mom relayed to me that she had taken him to see a psychologist recently but was disappointed. The psychologist said James had no clinical anxiety.

"He left the session covered in hives! How could the doctor not see that?" She asked.

Part of James's anguish was feeling that he should be able to lead a normal life. I assured him that his symptoms and the way he felt were real. But addressing them effectively was the puzzle. Many of my patients tried cannabis, and it didn't work for their intractable pain or insomnia. This was not unusual. Not only was James able to benefit from cannabis, but I felt he was conscientious enough to pursue his goals.

One technique would be to send him to a rehab center where he would be forced to quit cold turkey. But too often, this can result in replacing cannabis with a medication that may have failed already or has side effects that are just as debilitating as those of cannabis. Calling him a pot addict seemed too simple. He may have been addicted to the drug, but part of the addiction may have been to the very real benefits he received from using it. I ultimately felt that our work together was a failure, because he was not able to reduce his symptoms by changing to more effective antianxiety cannabinoids such as CBD. Because CBD is not euphoria inducing, it requires patience and dedication to fully understand how to utilize it. Many heavy cannabis users discount it as useless, because they can't feel its effects and lose patience before it builds up in the system, gaining efficacy and toning the nervous system toward balance.

James's quality of life stayed the same, and the drug that was helping him, cannabis, was probably harming his ability to grow. He is not alone. He still lives in his basement, smokes every day, plays Chopin, and continues to suffer from soul-crushing anxiety, remorse, depression, and regret about his situation.

Of Two Minds

James's suffering was real. But he is still lucky to live free of more serious mental diagnoses. Studies in recent years have shown the correlation between cannabis use and schizophrenia.[35] Many who start using cannabis early on later get a diagnosis of schizophrenia, which leads researchers to believe there is a link between smoking pot and becoming schizophrenic. The evidence points to a link, but individuals, as well as the ingestion methods, strains, and doses taken are different. I have seen patients in my consultation practice who were diagnosed with the disease but effectively used cannabis to regulate it where other drugs failed. And I have seen schizophrenic patients for whom cannabis seems to exacerbate their symptoms. I turned their request for cannabis down, as I was not comfortable with the idea that it might be contributing to their disease.

Many studies detailing the harms of cannabis—especially ones that claim it causes us to lose our sense of reality—are suspect to those who have been safely using the drug for decades. One major conundrum in the schizophrenia debate is that although there has been an increase in access to cannabis, an increase in numbers of smokers, and an increase in the potency of the drug, the rates of psychiatric disorders have not increased significantly in recent decades.[36] With inane antidrug commercials associating the effect of drugs on the brain with that of an egg frying in a skillet, the informed citizenry is suspicious when any scientific studies point to the psychiatric harms of cannabis. We become legitimately skeptical. But disorders of the mind are serious, and cannabis has a strong effect on the mind.

My professional opinion is that if you have been diagnosed with schizophrenia, or if it runs in your family, you should be very circumspect in using cannabis. According to a survey on the evidence, the correlation between schizophrenia and cannabis points to "the magnitude of cannabis exposure, suggesting a dose-response relationship."[37] The more pot you use, the higher the correlation to schizophrenia. People diagnosed with schizophrenia do seem to have a strong connection to cannabis. Nearly half of schizophrenic patients surveyed in one study were found to have used cannabis in the past year.[38] A comprehensive study published in 2007 by *Experimental Neurology* summarizes it well: "[In] individuals with an established psychotic disorder, cannabinoids can exacerbate symptoms, trigger relapse, and have negative consequences on the course of the illness. Exposure to cannabinoids in adolescence confers a higher risk for psychosis outcomes in later life and the risk is dose-related. However, it should be remembered that the majority of individuals who consume cannabis do not experience any kind of psychosis. There is a connection, we just don't know whether one is causing the other."[39]

I would go as far as to say that patients with a psychotic order should not use cannabis regularly, but when symptoms become greater than the side effects of drugs, sometimes persistent cannabis use—what we'd call chronic use—is effective treatment. One study of schizophrenic patients found that although a control group of healthy patients performed better on psychological tests, "within the schizophrenia group, a larger proportion of participants with lifetime cannabis abuse/dependence demonstrated better performance than those without lifetime abuse/dependence on a component of psychomotor speed. Frequency and recency of cannabis use were also associated with better neuropsychological performance, predominantly in the domains of attention/processing speed and executive functions."[40] Since other drugs can harm the psychiatric patient as well, one way to think about the evidence is that cannabis, like pharmaceuticals, is capable of harming and helping. Science is still working on it. It becomes less a question of objective scientific study and more a subjective decision made by the patient, his or her caretakers, and health practitioners.

When it comes to using cannabis for diseases of the mind, a more subjective or holistic approach might be helpful. There is no one-size-fits-all drug or treatment for a person who has had a break from reality. These patients are, by definition, not sharing our reality, so to assume we have the answer to "correcting" their mind may be invalidating at the very least. I deeply empathize with patients and families dealing with mind imbalances of any form. The root of the word "schizophrenia" is "split mind." The patient is of *two minds*. Put this way, it is a disease most of us should be able relate to. All brains are literally split into two independent hemispheres. Being of two minds *is* the state of our mind. Some split-brain experiments point to the idea that each of the two sides has its own consciousness.[41] This is a dichotomy many teenagers (and adults) can relate to when they think of their own consciousness and that of their parents. Subjectively, it is debatable which side is "correct" because reality is subjective, consciousness is subjective, and the mental effects of cannabis are subjective. This makes things complicated. I am not saying we should disregard the expertise of professionals or parents, but when treating diseases of the mind, all parties must acknowledge that subjectivity and perception are at work when it comes to drugs that alter the mind.

Drug companies have created pharmaceuticals to address psychosis and schizophrenia. Many of the drugs are effective, bringing stability and normalcy to the patient. Many of the drugs, as I mentioned earlier in the chapter, are also associated with violent acts and sustaining psychosis.[42] I met many patients diagnosed with schizophrenia who felt betrayed by "arrogant" doctors who prescribed debilitating medication after a hurried office visit. Sometimes the process of weaning themselves from the medication, as well as overcoming the side effects, took years of their lives. I've also met patients whose parents admitted them to psychiatric wards because they caught them flushing their pills down the toilet and smoking pot instead. In the hospital, they are dosed up on more meds, which exacerbate the disconnect from reality, their parents, and health providers. As with many "problem cases," in the medical field, psychiatric patients might also feel isolated and shamed on top of experiencing the symptoms associated with their disease. Doctors who have a thousand patients on their roster and whose brains are most comfortable in the materialistic reality of medical school, clinical settings, and pharmaceutical salesmen, can often be of little help to the patient who has struggled mentally and emotionally to navigate the world. Mental health is a complex societal challenge, but putting patients in jail for consuming, buying, or growing a plant that may help them is a poor solution.

Within the framework of medicinal cannabis, there is a potential solution that I believe could be a barometer of patient progress and stability. Aspirin is derived from willow bark, but rarely do we go out to a willow tree when we have a headache and grind some bark down to make a homemade aspirin. Few PhD's in chemistry would attempt to formulate any one of the thousands of drugs on the market. It is a well-established industry with complex research and development. But the culture of wanting a pill for every ailment disconnects millions from a natural, personal responsibility–based approach to their health. Medical cannabis, however, can be homegrown. Having a personal relationship with the production of their medicine can give people agency.

The sixty-seven plants and dozens of jars of remedies that were taken from my home served more than two hundred patients. The garden and processing space required for an operation that size was just over a third of my basement. A single patient, especially one with a continual need for a supply of cannabis medicine, needs far less space. In just a few hours a week, a patient can grow and maintain an indoor garden suitable for his or her medicinal needs. Plants need light, water, nutrients, and someone who can deliver these ingredients effectively enough to sustain a healthy garden.

If the garden is thriving, with the patient taking full responsibility, could this be a sign that the patient is also thriving? Obviously, some patients are physically unable to move, let alone tend a garden. But if the garden is failing because the patient *won't* get off the couch long enough to go water the plants, then maybe the patient needs to think more deeply about health and why he is using cannabis or other medications. Many physically disabled patients tend their own gardens successfully. Able-bodied patients should be able to do the same. There is no prescription for a cannabis garden. Most states with medical marijuana laws allow for some home growing. A patient who has spent hours tending a pot garden may have far more expertise growing weed in his basement than a PhD in horticulture would. Some growing methods are simple and some are complex. But what a patient can create is a closed loop of medication production and consumption. If a patient wants to maintain supply, he has to monitor his use and care for the garden.

I am neither providing a scientific solution to the conundrum of perceived versus diagnosed disorders of the mind nor suggesting that being a successful pot grower is a true indicator of a patient's mental health and stability. A trial could conceivably be done to test my hypothesis, but results will ultimately be based on the perception of the patient, his or her loved ones, and the professionals advising the family medically.

Many patients are already growing cannabis and literally reaping the benefits. They grow their herbal medicine and manage their psychiatric or physical symptoms by experimenting with different strain varieties and processing methods. Some patients not only can reduce their pharmaceutical intake but can derive a deeper, more spiritual and therapeutic relationship with the medicine that nurtures them. Just as we are ultimately responsible for our health, we have to be responsible for the other organisms living in our home. We have to feed and shelter them. We have to raise them and show them love if we want love in return. For decades, patients who suffer from mental and physical disorders have secretly grown cannabis, because humans require a wide variety of options for treatment. They may take pills, but they also take their health into their own hands by growing this nervous system–regulating plant. I hear the following sentiment from patients all the time: "My doctor was amazed by my progress. I of course didn't tell him that I was using cannabis. He just told me to keep doing whatever I was doing because it was working."

These are the patients who are secretly using cannabis. Anyone who enjoys eating the tomatoes she's lovingly grown on her back porch can only imagine the empowerment a patient must feel who has increased his own quality of life with his homegrown cannabis. Just as caring for a pet can give elderly people purpose and joy, growing marijuana can get sick people up in the morning. It gets their hands in the dirt and gives them a luscious garden to look at in the middle of winter. It gives them access to light and nature if they live in a dingy apartment building. It's been shown that artificial light therapy,[43] as well as having living plants around,[44] can reduce seasonal affective disorder. The first draft of the U.S. Constitution mandated that citizens grow hemp. I don't believe citizens should be *mandated* to grow medical marijuana, but certainly they should be *allowed* to grow it.

five

The Cannabis Householder

Although it is important for alternative medicine to have data to back up its efficacy, and for cannabis to be properly tested for contaminants, legislatures would do well to recognize that humans are part of nature and they seek out practitioners and therapies that make them feel connected. Here is a letter in support of the holistic aspect of medical cannabis that one of my patients sent to the district attorney during my legal case:

Dear Hampshire County District Attorney,

Due to medical privacy concerns, and the current stigma associated with cannabis, I must remain anonymous. I am a 49-year-old woman who was diagnosed with invasive ductal carcinoma in July 2013. I underwent a mastectomy on my left side, did sixteen weeks of dose-dense chemotherapy, and underwent six weeks of daily radiation treatments.

During my medical treatment, after surgery, and through some of the other treatments, I had to use opioids for pain, which I do not tolerate well (horrible constipation, bleeding hemorrhoids as a result). What I have learned from someone else, who lost his wife to a brain tumor, is that cannabis works on different pain receptors than opioids. Obviously, cannabis is far less addictive.

I have never been fond of cannabis so I did feel cautious about trying it. However, I had also read on the National Cancer Institute website that cannabis could reduce tumors, so I was eager to find a strain that was high in CBD—cannabidiol—as opposed to THC. The doctor had suggested to me that cannabis could also help my issues with anxiety and sleep problems. At the time that I met Ezra I was also taking an additional medication for helping me with sleep. The doctor also indicated that cannabis could be helpful for my irritable bowel syndrome.

Ezra was knowledgeable, articulate, obviously loved gardening and the growing process. He also made high-quality products with healthy delivery systems like coconut oil. I did not want to smoke or vaporize and he offered other options. I knew that he was a fully organic gardener, which was very important to me because I am also an organic gardener and grow a lot of my own food in a community garden. Knowing the person who was actually growing what I was ingesting was extremely comforting.

I am very concerned about having to go to a large dispensary where I am fearful that I will not know if I am getting appropriate products. I do not know if the people there will be as knowledgeable. I am worried that the dispensary will be crowded with lines, an unpleasant experience.

Ezra has been providing an extremely valuable service and I was dismayed to discover that he had been raided and charged after the enormous public service that he has been providing so many people in the community. I am saddened that the plant varieties which helped my IBS, sleep, and cancer symptoms are lost forever. When so many people are dying from opioid addiction, it is really heartbreaking to see someone like Ezra having all his carefully cultivated medicine destroyed.

Sincerely,
[Anonymous]

Finding a Seed

The legalization of marijuana has allowed many patients to gain access to a viable medicine for their ailments. But the inherent culture of intimacy between grower and consumer that marijuana prohibition has created over the generations has merits. Before legalization, many users had to develop trust, intimacy, and understanding with their dealer or grower. They were able to talk about what ailed them privately and were perhaps allowed to tour the garden where their medicine was produced. Growers and dealers who wanted to be successful cared about their customers and sought remedies that helped because their personal reputation was at stake. The term "big marijuana" has been coined to denote the giant, corporate culture vying for market share since legalization. But unlike the pharmaceutical industry, big marijuana doesn't have exclusive access or specific insight into growing and churning out the drug. A basement gardener can produce cannabis of quality equal to or higher than the most technologically advanced cultivator can in growing thousands of plants. The patients who have been chewed up and spit out of the similarly corporate culture of hospitals and modern medicine are often looking for healers and medicinal practitioners they can trust on an intimate level. Many friends, neighbors, and family members are already trusted by patients. And many of them know how to garden. If we're worried about big marijuana invading our communities and eroding that trust, then these individuals have the power to bring medicine to those they care about on their own.

A home gardener in possession of a single cannabis seed, if it is female, can produce a marijuana plant that can be turned into an infinite number of marijuana offspring, all of which, if treated properly, can be fifteen feet tall and produce over a pound of marijuana. This female plant does not need a male plant to produce hundreds of new seeds, either. If manipulated or "stressed" appropriately, the female plant begins to produce its own seeds.

A single female seed could also repopulate the entire planet with cannabis, because once grown, its branches can be sliced off and rooted, creating more plants. This process is called "cloning." A cut branch is a clone of its mother plant. It is how growers sustain specific strains in perpetuity. If the branch is cut and rooted before the plant begins to flower, the "mother" plant can then be flowered, finishing its life cycle.

For the readers who've made it this far in the story and still feel marijuana should be eradicated from the earth, you're pretty much out of luck. It is not necessarily easy to grow marijuana commercially, but unlike other illegal drugs like cocaine and opium, cannabis can grow anywhere.

Cloning does increase the complexity of the cannabis garden, but if a person wants to reproduce those precise genetics, cloning has to be perfected. Thousands of unique strains are lost every year to growers finishing out a plant's life cycle without cloning it—or, in thousands of other cases like my own, by police officers throwing the strains away. There are already tens of thousands of varieties of cannabis, so it's not a big loss for the recreational cannabis industry. But since every strain is different, could a discarded one be holding the key to resolving an individual's chronic pain, anxiety, or brain tumor? Many growers share strains with friends for this reason. If you lose it or get raided, a friend will safely keep the genetics for future generations. Some strains of cannabis have no original seed form and exist only as clones. They are shared from grower to grower over the generations.

If you can't get a clone from a friend (or online group dedicated to growing), an online seed bank is a simple option. Any basic Internet search will uncover the dozens of seed companies online selling thousands of strains of marijuana. For some would-be growers, the war on drugs is so pervasive in their minds that they fear conducting a mere Internet search for cannabis seeds will bring the SWAT team to their door. Therefore, they feel safer seeking seeds through friends or gathering them from the weed they smoke.

Technically, possessing a cannabis seed is not illegal, because it neither carries enough THC to be deemed contraband nor has yet produced a cannabis plant. Thus the seed companies, all outside the United States, get away with what they do by providing a warning on their Web sites: *Purchasing cannabis seeds is for souvenir purposes only. Seeds are not intended for cultivation.* Then, they go into detail about the best medium to grow them in, how long the plants need to flower before harvest, what size they will grow to indoors or out, and ultimately, how the high feels when you are finished growing your "souvenir" and roll it into a joint. The plethora of online seed banks is one of many legal marijuana loopholes—like head shops selling bongs for "*tobacco products only*"—that keep law enforcement scratching its head and the cannabis economy growing.

At an online seed bank, you will find photographs depicting the flowers on a mature cannabis plant after the seed has reached fruition. If you don't know what you're looking for, most of the photographs look identical. Typically, the image focuses on the flower or bud of the plant at the tail end of its four-month life cycle, framed by a black background to make the colors pop out. To a cannabis connoisseur, it is the botanical equivalent of a Playboy centerfold, the female flower bursting forth and displaying its pumped-up genitalia in hopes of collecting a speck of male pollen. Sadly for her, unless the grower is a strain breeder or seed producer, pollen-producing males are detrimental to a pot garden. Pollen makes seedy buds and seeds make for headaches when you smoke them. Seed banks usually offer what is called "feminized seeds," which reduce the chance that a male will propagate from them. Male seeds still occur. I have been called in to assess a client's strangely forming cannabis plants in late summer or, if grown indoors, late in the flowering cycle. Instead of rotund, sticky buds, the plants have little testicle-like bulbs hanging down from where the branches meet the main stalk. Males and females essentially look identical before the flower stage, but if you catch a male plant before its pollen sacks explode, it can be safely removed from a garden without seeding female flowers. The leaves of a male plant can be brewed into a light anointing oil—altering the end-of-life symptoms of a person like David in chapter 2—but it contains very little in the way of medicinal cannabinoids.

Then there are the strain names. Disappointingly, the culture of naming strains seems to reflect the low-consciousness culture of illicit cannabis more than what the strain can do for the conscientious user. A name such as Train Wreck may help explain what it does to one's consciousness, but it's not particularly useful in determining its medicinal subtleties. Here are the "A" strains from a single medical marijuana Web site, now defunct.

A Train	Accidental Tourist	Alaskan Thunderfuck
AK 47	Alaskan Ice	Apollo 13
Alien Dawg	Andys Ak-47	Agent Orange
Abra Cadabra	Afghan Kush	Alien Blues
AK47 x Skunk	Alaskan Thunder	Arizonan Assassin
Alien Dream	Bolt	OG
Acapulco Gold	Anthrax	AK 46
AK48 Amnesia	Afgooey	Australian Blue

Medical marijuana was not on my radar when I started to grow it, but intuitively I felt that avoiding names like AK-47 and Anthrax would be a more civilized place to start. As I discovered the miraculous medicinal properties of some strains, I cringed to think of a little old lady asking for Anthrax (or Alaskan Thunderfuck, for that matter) at a dispensary to ease her ailments. For all the potheads' paranoia about law enforcement, naming strains after a terrorist's weapon seemed like a government surveillance red flag waiting for attention: "*Sir, you may want to take a look at this. Some guy is talking about growing his own Anthrax!*"

Going by the purported ease of growing, the plant's small overall stature, and my exhaustion from searching the possibilities, I went with a strain called Early Misty: six seeds for ninety bucks. It's expensive, but once you realize that those six seeds could provide an unlimited amount of product and income for the well-schooled gardener, $90 seems cheap. I also realized that strains are not identical if grown in different environments. I traded plants with other growers whose end result looked and felt different from my original strain. We could tell that it was the same strain, but each choice in the growing process alters the cannabinoid and terpene profile. I realized that once I began growing a strain, it was molecularly unique, and therefore I could change the name to better reflect its medicinal effect. For example, I changed a strain named Bubblegum to Twilight because it was good for relaxing in the evening and combating insomnia. A White Widow strain became Golden Mind for its ability to inspire creativity and ease depressive thoughts. (My client who rediscovered nature photography after her leg amputation broke her creative block with this strain.) A strain named Affie became Affection because it seemed to enhance compassion and emotional connection. My OG Kush strain became River Stones because its hard, round buds caused a deeply sedative effect. It is important for data collection to keep track of a genetic line or original name of a cannabis strain, but once it is in your garden, you can call it whatever you want. A genetic test is the true determinant of its lineage.

Growing Marijuana in One Easy Step

I tell people that yes, cannabis grows like a "weed," but only in the most ideal conditions. Many people will say it is very easy to grow. Others try it and never manage to keep a plant alive. Some who grew pot in their youth will pronounce that prices are a rip-off because they once grew it in college. "It's not hard to do," they scoff. What is difficult about growing cannabis is sustaining a high-quality harvest, month after month, without mechanical error, pests, drought, mold, nutrient burn, crop failure, or getting arrested. If you're thinking of growing in your home, you can rest assured that the vast majority of marijuana growers never get caught. A map of all the clandestine gardens across the country would reveal a shocking number of basement, attic, garage, and backwoods grows. There are tens of thousands of people growing pot in their homes, as they have been for decades, often unbeknownst to the very family members living with them. With the proper light and ventilation, plants can be grown in bathrooms, closets, dorm rooms, cupboards, and even desk drawers. A clandestine marijuana grow may be the reason your neighbor always seems to have a new car parked in his driveway. If you are a parent who discovers your teen's garden in a closet, then rest assured that he or she is far in advance (at least in terms of horticultural discipline) of your average pot smoker.

Legislatures, departments of public health, and concerned communities that know little about the plant are doing their best to regulate this living organism in states where laws are evolving. As noted earlier, they restrict the number of plants that can be grown or the location of legal marijuana grow operations. Regulating plant count has always been a baffling approach to me. A single pot plant can fit in the palm of your hand and another can be as large as a horse. If you restrict the number of plants citizens can grow, what size plant will they choose? The Drug Enforcement Agency, according to its Web site, proudly eradicated over four million marijuana plants in 2014.[1] But that's just the ones that were found. The ones that are missed literally go up in a puff of smoke. Legislatures and those who are familiar only with the drug stereotypes forget that this drug is a living organism. As long as seeds will grow in dirt, citizens will grow their own pot. Citizens who have the most to lose from getting caught buying it on the street grow their own.

I tell clients that if they want to be successful growing marijuana, they should start with the step that is the most comfortable to them. Growing marijuana is as complicated as you want it to be. If you are not attached to the results, you can put a seed in some dirt under a fluorescent light bulb for a couple months and with a little water, you will have a delightful specimen bringing joy and adoration. You won't have much in the way of consumable product, but at least you will have established a relationship with your plant. It will be two months of silently gazing at your baby (a huge time suck) and perhaps hours of reading grow help forums online, perusing cannabis growing books, and investigating techniques at the local hydroponic store. "Hydroponic" refers to a type of growing that generally uses nonsoil growing mediums, such as highly aerated water. Hydroponic lettuce is common at the supermarket. It's a grow method that can be modularized and expanded, is often done indoors, and therefore cannabis growers and hydroponics growing go hand in hand. Pot growers use soil indoors as well, but a *hydroponic* or *hydro* garden store has become a euphemism for a marijuana grow store. Owing to the fact that few people have ever met another person who grows a legitimately hydroponic crop at home, the *hydroponic* store in your town most likely has a customer base of primarily pot growers.

For the sake of preserving the culture and community they have quietly nurtured over the years, you should not go into a hydro store and ask if the owners can help you grow marijuana. Depending on the local laws, they will probably say no, because to do so would be conspiring to break federal law. But the person behind the counter will have an uncanny knack for growing, cloning, and flowering indoor "tomatoes." Once you have established yourself in the hydro store, namely by skirting around cannabis nomenclature as you ply store employees with questions, as I did, then you realize that these dudes are masters of their craft and have little time for the sniggering customers who wink and say the "M" word out loud.

If you know how to sprout seeds a certain way, then do it that way. If you are used to growing things on your windowsill in the summer, then start like that. The plant, if you find yourself drawn to nurturing green things, will give you plenty of time to discover the next step that makes sense for you. With each mistake made, a new lesson is learned. Attachment to results breed disappointment. I entered it as a gardener, not as an underground cannabis user. The prohibition on marijuana has made people so obsessed about getting the most from their high-value grow that they sweat every last detail. It's important to remember that it's just a plant.

Growing outside is also fun, as long as it is legal to do so or the helicopters can't see your plants. As cannabis follows the same life cycle of any annual plant, a seed or plant can go into the ground around June 1 and be harvested in early October. Growers produce fifteen-foot-tall specimens by growing them large under lights first, and then transplanting them outside.

Questions inevitably arise as one grows. Often, the solution is simple. But it's the parsing through the contrary information online or at the hydro store that can be difficult. I discovered how opinionated growers could be in my early visits to my local hydroponic store.

"What do you guys recommend for a nutrient brand?" I asked an employee stocking shelves.

"ProGrow, 100 percent. I used Green Time for a couple years and it sucked. Then I went with OrganiGrow and had some monster crops until it started burning all my leaves. They changed the formula or something. I'm using ProLine now and it's the best, hands down. Best harvests I've ever had." He pointed rapidly to the three brands among dozens on the shelf. I found that the labels were overly colorful, rarely told me what they were specifically used for, and appeared to be designed by someone under the influence of a mind-altering drug of some sort.

Essentially, all the brands have a "grow" product, a "bloom" or flowering product, and various other additives that their brand loyalists can't live without. There's rarely anything on the side of the bottle to differentiate between the nutrient lines or their ingredients. It's only required to list the ratios of nitrogen, phosphorous, and potassium in the nutrient solution. More nitrogen means it's better for the vegetative (or early summer) stage. More potassium and phosphorous generally means it's better for the flowering (or late-summer) stage. But the ratio and percentage are different in each nutrient, causing more head scratching. It's rather mysterious how so many brands can make it onto the shelves.

Okay, I thought. This guy seems to know what he's talking about.

"Dude, no way," said a fellow customer who came closer, unable to ignore our conversation. He was big, wearing a bowling shirt with the name Mort on it, and had multiple neck tattoos going up toward his bald head. His burly arm was holding a two-and-a-half-gallon bucket of a fertilizer additive named Atomic Bud Explosion. (This amount of fertilizer could have fed my lone plant for about three years.) The graphic on the side of the bottle displayed a mushroom cloud exploding out of a garden row. All cannabis fertilizer imagery is in metaphor, as the fertilizer companies that populate the hydroponic industry can't tell you that their product was developed for a certain illegal plant.

He went on. "I wouldn't touch ProLine. One, it's not organic, so unless you want your 'tomatoes' to taste like chemicals, then don't buy it. Two, their ratios are way off. That shit will burn your plants. CannaBurst is the best line, hands down. They actually grow real 'tomatoes' with it in Holland, if you know what I mean. So they know their shit."

Okay, this guy seemed more convincing. He wasn't a salesman. He was a real grower. And "Canna" was in the name, so that made sense. I nodded humbly in agreement.

The employee responded, "Yeah, but CannaBurst is twice as expensive for basically the same exact ingredients. It's only because of the name. People fall for 'C-a-n-n-a' and think they're getting some superior product. Besides, they're so 'organic' that plants can't even uptake their nutrients because half of the shit isn't soluble in water. It's all in chunks at the bottom."

They weren't exactly fighting. It was more of a debate two scientists would have over a theory that hasn't been tested yet. Okay, yes, the employee is going to know his stuff, I thought. I should go with his suggestion, but the guy with the huge bottle appeared to be a professional pot grower. The conversation went through a half dozen other chemical, horticultural, and soil science topics, until I eventually retreated to the checkout counter. I decided to skip my nutrient purchase until the next time I came in; no need to offend one of the passionate experts by choosing the wrong product. When I finally left, they had moved on from parts per million of trace elements to the authenticity of nutrient brand founders. Eventually, I found a ma and pa hydroponic store where the owners were warm and approachable.

Regardless of what brand, grow store culture, or cultivation method you choose, the process can be extremely rewarding. After discovering that I could provide my own opinions on the subject in a less confrontational way, I had a client come to me for growing advice. His newly acquired medical marijuana card entitled him to cultivate ten ounces of medical marijuana every two months. He had spent years buying cannabis to help his mood swings, many of which were fueled, ironically, by the deep fear and paranoia he felt that he might be arrested. He was in his late fifties, a shy and gentle man who lived alone in a low-income apartment. He had asked me if I would show him my basement garden, and although it's an unwritten law in the grower culture to never show your garden to a stranger, I relented. When I brought him downstairs and unzipped my grow tent, revealing the sea of green and warm yellow glow, he doubled over, seemingly in pain.

"I'm sorry," he said. He grabbed my arm to help pull himself up. "It's just so beautiful. I've never seen a living marijuana plant in person before. I'm crying right now."

We were both sober. They were just plants. But I empathized. It's deeply emotional for many people who have had to hide their passion their entire lives. For medical marijuana patients, the act of caring for a medicinal plant that eases their aches and pains, PMS, or fibromyalgia is a reciprocal and therapeutic relationship that the pharmaceutical industry will never understand. Sure, pot growers are often "just trying to get high," but hydro stores are full of passionate, intelligent, and driven gardeners who are bringing into the world a plant that has meaning to them far beyond the pot stereotypes or tiny pills their doctors are prescribing.

Selecting a Plant for Its Effect

Years into deepening my own relationship with cultivating marijuana, I sat down for a consult with a middle-aged guy named Will. A part-time social worker by trade, inspired by the article about me in the paper, he was clearly heartfelt about all things marijuana, and he was determined to enter the industry as I had. I told him about my practice, and he bounced business ideas off of me, as he was primarily there to network.

Will was an educated man in his early fifties. He was more of a shaggy, gray-haired type with hiking boots and flannel shirt than your typical white-collared professional, but he was burned out on social work and wanted a new career. I could tell that he probably spent more time smoking and dreaming up ideas than actually implementing them, but I gave him the benefit of the doubt. He asked me the perennial question of what I thought about specific strains and their effect on people.

"What do you think is the best strain that you've seen for like, headaches?" he asked.

"Well, I think the idea that a single strain can be a miracle cure for a single ailment is a bit of a misconception. I know there are people who swear by their one strain for their symptom, but it is unlikely that that same strain will have the same effect on another person, let alone thousands of people, consistently." I had seen the Web sites that rated the strains based on their effects: euphoria, pain relief, sedation, body versus head high, and so forth. The ratings are unscientific on many levels. For example, few people know if the "Kush" strain they're smoking is the same "Kush" strain someone is smoking across the country or across campus—or even across the hall. One's experience of a strain is also very subjective. Is the strain working for the ailment on a physiological level? Or is the user merely feeling better about the ailment as the cannabis provides an effective distraction from the symptom? Do all the strains they try work the same, or is it a strain-specific effect? What was the method of ingestion? How "ripe" was the flower before it was picked? What was the cure time? What were they *told* the effects were going to be? Was it smoked in a bong or a vaporizer? The variables go on and on.

"Ultimately the best way to determine if a strain is good for a certain ailment is for a patient to work with a caregiver or dispensary that supplies a consistent product and then take good notes on the effect it has on symptoms. Medical marijuana, done correctly, requires due diligence on the part of the patient. There's no miracle strain for one ailment, across the board," I said.

"Yeah, that's true," said Will. "But what I want to do is to really discover that perfect strain for each problem, you know. Wouldn't it be amazing if you could just know, okay, this strain works for cramps. This one works for shoulder pain. This one is for neuropathy. That's what I want to do."

I was experiencing déjà vu. "It's a cool idea, Will, but it's akin to what the conventional medical model is trying to do. It isolates an ailment from the person and tries to just solve it with a discrete molecule. Then they've created another pill they can produce en masse that helps a percentage of people and doesn't help others. Sometimes it makes patients worse. It means doctors can talk less to patients and prescribe more pills. I don't personally think that cannabis will go in as precise a direction if it hasn't been able to already. Many people still think its medical benefits are a hoax, yet it's been medically legal in California since 1996. I think various strains have various effects on each person's metabolism, physiology, mood, and the attitude they project onto their illness. Yes, cannabis has bona fide science to back it up. It definitely helps with pain, with sleep, with nausea, appetite, et cetera. But not everybody, and certainly not every strain that helps a person sleep, will help all people sleep."

"Yeah, that's true. Man, I love your approach, man. It's so cool what you are doing. I totally agree. The pharmaceutical companies just want to shove pills down your throat, but cannabis is a much better medicine."

"For some people, yes. Cannabis is not that different than many conventional meds. Some people love how Percoset or Vicodin 'feels,' and some people can't tolerate it. They've actually done placebo studies on different-sized placebo pills. They figured out that bigger sugar pills tend to do better for certain symptoms than smaller sugar pills!"[2]

"No shit?" said Will.

"It's true, and it's crazy. I think the point is that the mind is a powerful tool, and cannabis, in conjunction with the right framing of the mind, can provide more options for health."

"Yeah, that's true. My girlfriend used Percoset for pain once, and she hated it. That's why I think it would be awesome if you could find the right strain that just worked perfectly for pain. And then you just sell that strain to people with pain, you know. I think that would be really cool."

"Yes, I hear you—but like I said—I'm not sure cannabis works that way. I'm not sure opioids even work that way. That's why there are so many different opioids. People need different things. People need to be guided and need to do their own due diligence to discover what works for them."

If you're like Will, you might find that it doesn't really matter what strain you choose, as you can't remember what the last one felt like. A friend of mine who is an astrophysicist likes to smoke in the evenings and then ponder his mathematical computations for finding exoplanets thousands of light years away. I assumed he'd be a good person to tell me what he thought of the different strains I produced.

"I get the idea *intellectually* that they are different, and at first I think I have a sense of it. But five minutes in I'm so wrecked that I can't tell the difference one way or the other," he told me.

This may be true for your average smoker, as determining a strain's effects on a nonailing body can be elusive. But a patient dealing with an acute symptom knows when a strain or product is working and when it is not.

Indica versus Sativa

There is one aspect of strain selection that I believe is important for a patient to know from the start: the difference between sativa and indica. As I have referenced throughout the book, a sativa strain of cannabis describes an effect that is stimulating and is generally considered to be a mind-oriented or wakeful high. Indica describes cannabis that is sedative and felt in the body. If you can never remember the difference between sativa and indica, then this mnemonic might help: *indica is indicated for nights and sativa is indicated for Saturday nights.*

The shape of a mature, female cannabis flower is reminiscent of the wavy top of a soft-serve ice cream cone, with fuzzy green hairs and a frosting of cannabis trichomes. Trichomes are the sticky, microscopic balls of cannabinoid-filled resin and terpenes that plants are bred to produce en masse. A long, slender ice cream–shaped flower indicates sativa attributes. Squat, round ice cream cone shapes tend toward indica effects.

There are other discerning physical characteristics that help differentiate sativa and indica. Wide, short leaves on a cannabis plant tend to denote an indica strain. Long, skinny leaves can signify a stimulating or sativa strain. When it comes to sedating or stimulating a user, sativa and indica are extremely important. But the difference between sativa and indica from a scientific perspective is still unsettled. Biologists who have looked into it can't determine any genetic patterns in these plants. Some say differences between sativa and indica are a farce, as their genetic markers are untraceable.[3] Thus, they believe that labeling a strain as sativa or indica is not an accurate way to tell a plant's objective effects. Although the science may not yet be able to locate sativa and indica in the genetic code and consistency of effect from person to person is unpredictable, the distinction is not a farce. Cannabis users and professionals like myself have observed the connection between plant physiology and medicinal outcome. With a few exceptions (such as the Pennywise in chapter 2), I have found that my sativa plants produce consistently sativa effects and indica plants produce consistently indica results. Hybrid plants with a spectrum of sativa and indica traits also produce a spectrum of results. It will be mapped out scientifically in a matter of time. Currently, since it doesn't fit into the scientific model, we can shed light on this disparity from an ancient cannabis perspective—that of Ayurvedic medicine. Through the lens of Ayurveda, the effects and difference between sativa and indica become more commonsense.

In Ayurveda, there are three main body types or *doshas* that help practitioners diagnose and treat imbalances in the human body. They are similar to the concept of ectomorph, endomorph, and mesomorph in describing physiology. But Ayurveda extrapolates these concepts beyond just the physical to personality and behavior as well. The *vata dosha* refers to a physique that is tall and slender: that is, an ectomorph. Often, the personality of a *vata* individual is described as talkative, creative, and flighty. He or she might also be prone to anxiety. A *vata* individual may need a lifestyle that is calm, structured, and nourishing. I believe *vata* corresponds nicely with the concept of sativa. A sativa high is in the mind. It makes one wakeful and talkative. And it can provoke anxiety and worry in the user. The physiology of a sativa plant is also tall and slender, just like a *vata* person. Sativa plants have long, pointed leaves (like the fingers of ectomorphs), and their flowers are also elongated and airy. For someone who's anxious and tends to misplace his or her keys regularly, a sativa strain may not be recommended, because it will exacerbate unwanted symptoms. An indica strain may be just the thing to calm the *vata* person and provide a deep, nourishing sleep.

Indica, on the other hand, is represented well by the Ayurvedic *dosha* called *kapha*. *Kapha* describes an endomorphic body type that is dense and round, with thick fingers, big, full eyes, and a wide face. Indica cannabis plants have short, stubby leaves. They grow lower to the ground, with more leaf density than sativas, and their flowers are also round and bulbous. A *kapha* individual may be more sedentary, mellow, and prone to depression. As indica strains are sedative and calming, they may exacerbate the issues a *kapha* individual experiences. A sativa strain may be beneficial for *kapha* types who have difficulty getting motivated to exercise or freeing their minds from the doldrums. Sativas are also used to break one out of the torpor of a creative block or depressive state. They stimulate the creative mind and can provoke laughter, joy, and the desire to get out and move one's body.

A diverse cannabis garden will have an indica strain, a sativa strain, and a hybrid variety. Hybrids are described well by the third Ayurvedic *dosha: pitta. Pitta* is defined as a medium or mesomorphic body type. It leans toward neither slenderness nor rotundity. Plants from hybrid strains have a variety of indica and sativa traits. They are essential for the user who does not want to be too tired using an indica or too stimulated using a sativa. Some hybrids have long, lanky branches and round, dense flowers. Others grow low and bushy, but their leaves are thin and long. The effects of hybrids are just as diverse. Some inspire activity but prevent much thinking at all. Other hybrids enhance talking and brainstorming yet prevent the user from getting off the couch. All strains require experimentation and good note taking in order to understand the range of effects. (According to Ayurveda, humans are also diverse in that everyone contains a unique ratio of all three *doshas.*) When you intertwine a strain's potential effects with the endocannabinoid system of an individual who also has a range of physiological and personality traits, you begin to understand why there is a multitude of variables to consider.

The Grower's Dilemmas

The pot smokers you know or in the movies you watch may be forgetful. They may get out of bed at noon and eat junk food in front of the TV. But maintaining a quality cannabis garden in one's basement requires a certain level of discipline, fortitude, and gravitas. Like children, plants require the proper sustenance, environment, and care twenty-four hours a day, seven days a week, 365 days a year. You can, of course, design your garden system to function without constant vigilance, but like parenting, growing will require commitment. It also requires managing some unexpected circumstances. In Massachusetts, adults over twenty-one can grow up to twelve plants legally per household, and the cool temperatures of basements are ideal environments for growing cannabis under hot lights. But at the same time, basements often require access by random strangers. Living in a hundred-year-old house in New England has meant that my furnace and gas lines have needed repair almost every winter. One weekday morning on a subzero day, we woke up to find no gas coming out of our stove and only cold water available. I had no choice but to call the gas company.

"What about your plants?" My wife asked.

"I'll see when the gas company can come. I guess I'll just move them up to the attic until their service person is gone. I'll ask if they have to go into the basement at all. I assume they'll only need to thaw the line outside." I dialed the number at 7 a.m. Miraculously, the operator picked up right away.

"Sounds like you have a frozen gas line. Our guy is in your neighborhood already. He'll be there in ten minutes," she said hurriedly. Shocked by the brevity of the call, I had not considered a delaying tactic. She hung up.

"Fuuuuuck," I exhaled. I hoped he could fix it from the outside, but if not, my grow space was a few feet away from my furnace and gas water heater. I bolted downstairs and surveyed the area from the perspective of a repairman. I didn't have enough time to get the plants up to the attic and didn't want to be half finished when the gas company showed up. Besides, moving plants around wafts their terpenes in every direction. After a few calming breaths, I thought rationally. He is not going to be looking for a marijuana grow space. He'd be focusing on the gas problem, so I had to frame the area in a way that kept his eyes from drifting off. If he wasn't given the opportunity to question what the weird black tent with vent tubes coming out of it was, his mind wouldn't connect the dots. I gathered up three clip lights I had hanging in my work shop and hastily attached them to the exposed ceiling joists and plumbing in the basement ceiling. One pointed toward the furnace area from the right, one lit the water heater from the left, and one floodlight hung directly in front of the grow space, its light blackening the tent behind it. Then the doorbell rang.

"Yeah, we get about three calls a day from your neighborhood when temps get this low. The water condenses and freezes in the line. Gotta check the lines at your furnace, check them running into your basement, and restart the pilot lights." The repairman's massive, snowy boots clomped down my basement stairs toward my helpless plants. Knowing I had a plant so life altering in its legal status buried deep in my basement, while I led a 250-pound stranger directly to it, was a humbling experience. I wondered, as I did several times in similar circumstances before legalization, if it would be my last view of my basement, my last interaction with an unknown civilian until he called the cops and they took me away forever.

"Well, you're the neighborhood hero, then! Super appreciate you coming out so soon," I chirped. Guileless chitchat was all part of the illusion I was trying to project. He knelt down in front of the furnace and got to work, his back three feet from a Schedule I dangerous drug growing directly behind him. I handed him a foam pad I used when I was tending my plants.

"Feel free to use this for your knees," I said. Maybe he won't turn me in if I'm really nice.

"Hey, thanks. 'Preciate it. The knees do get kinda stiff," he replied.

When he came upstairs and clicked on the gas at the stove I knew I had made it. I bid him farewell at the front door with a sincere thank-you and warm smiles, allowing myself to surf happily on the receding wave of adrenaline. I was confident I wasn't going to jail. With each fooled repairman and disappearing garden trick, I became more emboldened and more convinced of my entitlement to grow the plant.

"Nobody gives a shit!" I would rant to my wife after a near miss, adrenaline and cortisol still coursing through my bloodstream. "It's ten plants growing in a box that nobody can see even when they're three feet from it. Why is this country so obsessed with eradicating marijuana? I'm not going to give it to kids. If I were brewing beer, I could offer one to the guy and he'd probably take it. He probably even smokes weed, but I'm sweating bullets walking him down there. Meanwhile, if I found out he smoked weed, he'd be terrified I'd get him fired. It's all so ridiculous!"

I eventually doubled the size of my garden, as well as my electric bill. "You are using 200 percent more energy on average than your most efficient neighbors," read the "home-use energy report" I received in the mail from the electric company. Seeing the raw evidence of my illegal activity on the page made my heart skip a beat. I could fool an occasional utility worker. But this was more serious.

I went into the grow forums online to see how others were dealing with the issue. I typed "energy report grow forum" into my browser and found conversations, conspiracies, and debates spanning years. I learned that using an inordinate amount of electricity in your home is not probable cause for a search or investigation. The electric company does not alert the police to shut down its best-paying customers. As long as you pay your bill, it is illegal for the utility company, as well as law enforcement, to search your home on the basis of your energy usage alone. If they are investigating you for a crime, they can subpoena the electric bill. Otherwise, you and other homeowners who run hot tubs, big computer servers, and indoor orchid gardens are all receiving similar home energy reports.

I also found the veil of my secret world parted on occasion by the conspicuously fragrant aspect of the cannabis plant. Luckily, the "hydroponic" gardening industry has sufficiently addressed the issue of the skunklike smell wafting through the neighborhood from indoor growing. There's a wide range of carbon filters, scent absorbers, and ionic odor neutralizers, all of which work. But when you are ready to harvest your crop, it is inevitable that the chopping, moving, and trimming of plants create fragrant airborne molecules that fill the house and drift outside. As when walking down the streets of a big city, one commonly catches a whiff of cannabis when walking by a cannabis-friendly home.

It was during a postharvest week that my wife had a close call. The unpredictability of who will catch the whiff can be hair-raising, as she experienced. My wife believed the laws were ignorant and outdated as well, but she did not find the close calls to be as philosophically invigorating as I did. On the fateful day, she was about to bring our children to their grandmother's house, along with a freshly baked apple pie. I had harvested the day before, and my plants were drying in the attic. One could smell the citrusy, earthy musk when walking by our house. I maintained that nobody would be alarmed unless he knew what he was smelling.

"If people recognize the smell, they'll be on our side. They'll probably enjoy it! Those who are foreign to it won't know what it is. I don't think it's an issue," I explained to friends who noticed the smell and worried about me. I found it particularly annoying that the scent of a plant could make people fearful and paranoid. But I'd had very little interaction with law enforcement. As she pulled out of the driveway, running a few minutes late, a police officer had walked from his parked cruiser toward her car door. Backing up, she hadn't seen him until he was upon her. She rolled the window down and the weed smell hovered between them in the early autumn air.

"Hello, officer. I'm sorry I didn't see you. Can I help you?"

"I'm sorry to bother you, ma'am. But we received a 911 call originating from this location and we wanted to confirm everything was okay," he said.

"Really? I don't know what that is about? I do live here, but I didn't make a 911 call!" She gave her most relaxed and unworried smile.

"Are you sure? We do have to respond to every call. But sometimes there are glitches," he replied.

"You're welcome to have a look around," she responded casually.

"No, that's okay. I'm sorry to bother you. Hey, what is that I smell—is that pie?" he asked.

"Uh—why, yes. Fresh apple pie right out of the oven. Bringing it to grandma's house!" She said cheerily.

"Well, I must say that that is the most delicious apple pie I have ever smelled. And two cute kids in the back. Aren't you three the picture of wholesome goodness! Sorry to bother you, ma'am."

"No problem, officer. Happy to help. Have a great day!"

I think I probably pushed the brush-with-police envelope as far as it would go before I pushed too far. To this day, although I empathize with the job law enforcement has in enforcing marijuana laws, I don't believe that the laws offer any net benefit to society, so the risks I took were worth it, in pushing society further toward a rational stance on the plant.

As I look back on the summer after I quit my teaching job, it was a romantic period. I had a lovely garden, a job at a garden store, and several individual clients. I went all out dressing up their gift bags, labeling the jars, and making their experience as high-end as possible. I had a little cannabis plant growing outside in my garden, free to sway in the breeze. It was Bubblegum, which evolved to become Twilight, after I had spent time assessing its effects. I would get my kids off to day camp, garden inside and out for a few hours, and have lunch on my back deck, so I could stare at the Twilight hidden among the lupine and butterfly bushes. I didn't have to grow a plant outside, but it seemed stupid not to. Why run electricity and eventually an air conditioner inside to create an artificial garden, when I had a real one in my back yard?

I also didn't have room for it in my grow tent, so on a whim, I planted the Twilight plant when it was six inches tall. Twilight was a beloved indica strain used for healthy digestion after dinner, increased libido, and a good night's sleep. It was early July, so I was sure it wouldn't get to be more than one or two feet tall. But by early August, before the flowers started showing, I cut a foot off the top branches to keep the height *under* three feet.

The plant was a fascinating experiment in visual cognition. For all intents and purposes, the Schedule I dangerous drug I was cultivating within a school zone in my back garden was hidden in plain sight. So ordinary was its presence among other, more flamboyant species, that without my pointing it out, no visitors ever noticed the plant. When I finally did point it out, its leaf shape was unmistakable.

I was overly confident in my illusion when a fence salesman came to our property to tell us about options for our dog. I knew he was coming and had our yard inspection route planned out to avoid direct contact with the Twilight plant. It was a beautiful summer day, so we chatted about our options on the back deck, the Twilight bush sitting quietly just fifteen feet away. Then, as I had planned, I walked him clockwise around the yard, starting from the opposite side of the deck. The plan was to walk the whole perimeter, and therefore we would miss the flower beds clumped together in the middle, near the house.

He was very clean cut, with a salesman's wink-and-smile demeanor. His starched polo shirt said "Chuck," and his short haircut was gelled just so. Chuck worked as a salesman for a corporation and had driven up from a conservative town about thirty minutes south. He was very friendly, but I still couldn't predict where he came down on the issue. If I had to guess, he probably never touched the stuff. Toward the end of our yard tour, he abruptly broke my planned trajectory.

"I can see the rest of the yard is self-explanatory, so no need to look over there," he said as he began to cut across my lawn back toward the deck and the paperwork he'd left on the picnic table. Two flower patches ahead would funnel him right past the now looming plant. I thought he would make it past without noticing, when he literally did a double take with his head and stopped short.

"Whu!? Uh, I know what that is—I almost walked right by it," he said, clearly shocked. I was silent. There was really no excuse for a four-foot-tall cannabis plant growing in the middle of my yard.

"You can't fool me! I've seen one of these before. I don't touch the stuff myself, but I actually have a funny story." My muscles eased up a bit, hoping it was a funny ha-ha story.

"My two buddies who—you know, smoke pot—well, they wanted to grow some one summer. They were too paranoid to do it at their house, so they asked *me* if I would put the plants in my backyard. Ask the guy who doesn't smoke the stuff, you know!? I didn't really care, though. I have a big backyard and the plants got big. I mean, they were like six feet high eventually. My buddies, man, they were so paranoid. They took care of them, and they were looking amazing. But they got so big that my buddies got too paranoid *to come over to my house!* They made *me* do all the work! Can you believe it?" he said.

"That is insane," I replied. Paranoid potheads avoiding arrest was not insane. It was insane that *this guy* grew their weed. It was insane that we were now standing next to my cannabis plant and he was telling me this story. I was flummoxed. Chuck went on.

"Well, at the end of the summer they went away for a couple weeks. They work together on the road doing line work. They told me to cut the plants down, let it dry, and put it into bags. So I went out there and chopped them down. I took all the leaves off and it filled like two big trash bags. It was a lot. I didn't know what I was doing, but I was pretty impressed with myself!"

"Wow," I said.

"Well, my buddies came back and I showed them the bags I had collected. They were like, 'Where's the tops?' 'What do you mean?' I said. They were like, 'Where's the flowers? The buds!?' Well, I have never even smoked pot once, so what did I know? When I cut them down I kept all the leaves—I thought that was the part they wanted! I recognized that part. I tossed everything else in the trash! That's what you get for making the square guy grow your marijuana!" He laughed.

"So don't worry or anything." He said, gesturing at my plant. We walked back over to the deck. Twilight's secret was safe with Chuck.

As laws evolve to deregulate the home cultivation of marijuana, the act of gardening at home will not induce so much paranoia, but issues will come up. Repairmen still have to enter basements, smells will still waft through the neighborhood, and kids will be observing their parents growing a plant that their school may still consider a federally illegal substance. But a small garden can provide enough cannabis remedies for the adults in a home, and it offers the opportunity for adults to have intelligent conversations with their children—and fence salesmen—about cannabis.

Everything in Moderation

A successful cannabis gardener will quickly find that a few plants can create far more cannabis and cannabis remedies than one knows what to do with. Many a middle-aged cannabis user may discover that his years of scraping out pipes and saving half-smoked joints is over, as he could never consume all of his crop. He now sweeps small buds and leaves up in his garden and throws them away, because already jars of the stuff fill the cupboards.

It is satisfying to finally feel one has enough quality cannabis that one doesn't have to hoard it or worry where it will come from, but overabundance does pose some problems. First, if an adult is in compliance with the law in Massachusetts, for example, then he or she can have about ten ounces of cannabis stored in jars at one time. One ounce can fit in a quart jar, so this is ten quarts of potent cannabis. The street value of ten ounces of cannabis at the time of this writing is about $2,500–$3,500. Ten ounces can make more than a gallon of potent oil. This much oil can produce over forty batches of brownies, enough for a block party in a major metropolis. Even if one makes a half gallon of oil and uses the other five ounces for smoking, it's still far too much cannabis per month for the average user. Many people could end up stoned all day, every day, if they consume it liberally. I know people who feel this is their preferred state of mind. And I know patients like Johnny in chapter 1, who need huge amounts of cannabis to keep the harder drugs at bay. But a balanced, healthy adult user does not need to be stoned all day—or at all, if she is merely looking for symptom relief. With cannabis intake, one has to decide one's own optimal amount. For some, it might be a few puffs in the evening, an edible ingested after a long day of work, or a few drops of topical oil applied to a sore neck. Others might find that a puff or two on the weekend is all their nervous system can handle. Any more makes their mind slow and foggy. More car keys are lost. Appointments are forgotten.

As with alcohol, sugar, and screen time, most people can tell when too much is bringing them out of balance and they need to ease off. Tolerance of THC increases over time, and some people find they require more of the drug to get the symptom relief they want. I have found with my clients that a forty-eight-hour break from cannabis can reset one's tolerance and bring down the quantity consumed. I also recommend weeklong or monthlong "cleanses" from cannabis (and other vices) in order to address cravings and reset one's awareness of use versus abuse. If you are on a spiritual path and want to strive to be your highest self, remember that *you can get high with cannabis, but you cannot get to your highest self.* Eventually, one's spirit needs room to grow without cannabis. I have made it my mission to help people along the whole spectrum of cannabis use for this reason. I know that with cannabis, quality of life can increase in the seriously ill who are already burdened by too many pharmaceutical pills. Cannabis can help guide them back to a life path that was lost. And I know that some cannabis users are burdened by too many puffs and have fallen off their potential path years ago. But I do believe there is a sweet spot for ingesting cannabis that will decrease pills and symptoms, increase quality of life, and maintain productivity and spiritual growth in the adult. For some it may mean growing the plant for a friend with cancer, but never ingesting it themselves.

The concept of spirituality is not a scientific one, but because cannabis alters consciousness, we have to consider metaphor in defining its medicinal use. The brain does not think in literal terms. Every thought pattern the brain forms is a *representation* of something—not the actual thing. Words are also a translation of the patterns in our brain. When we think of an apple, there is no apple in our brain. This simple yet baffling conundrum of objective reality is at the core of a heated debate in science, philosophy, and art: What is consciousness? In science, it is what is referred to as the "hard problem."[4] The problem is that they haven't found consciousness to be "stored" in the brain. It's not measurable or dissectible. But we all seem to agree that we have it.

Not only does cannabis contain compounds that affect our consciousness, our perception of the world, ourselves, and our ailments, but it also triggers cell behavior in the body of organisms that has been necessary for survival for hundreds of million years. The sum of all of these parts points to something bigger than what can be measured. Thus, the word "spirituality" is often brought up by practitioners of cannabis use who consider this synergy.

On the based of studies on the evolution of vertebrates, nematodes, and sea squirts,[5] it's thought that the endocannabinoid system has been in place in organisms for over five hundred million years.[6] As humans share a common ancestor with all organisms, five hundred million years ago was an era on the evolutionary tree when "we" were essentially much like plants ourselves. Scientists spend their entire careers trying to figure out where our physiology and plant origins end and our human consciousness begins. How does an animal perceive the world? Do plants have perception, taste, emotions? Are memories stored differently in the brains of different species? Why do people react differently to the same stimuli? Why do we all find a sunset beautiful? Do sea squirts find sunsets beautiful?

If we feel something crawling up our leg as we sit in the grass, we might experience a momentary panic as we brush the insect off, only to realize that it was a blade of grass tickling our skin. Consciousness is our physical awareness translated through the often-imaginative synapses of our brain. Embracing the full spectrum of consciousness, including what a cannabinoid-filled plant can offer, can give a patient hope. If I were trapped inside a broken body, plant consciousness is a form of consciousness I might want to embrace. Our subjective consciousness is also the reason we develop metaphors like yin and yang and indica and sativa in relation to curatives, or the smiley faces we see on the doctor's office wall that help us define our pain. There is also scientific evidence to back up a less limited and materialistic approach to medicine. In *Cure: The Journey into the Science of Mind over Body,* the author Jo Marchant sums up her findings as follows: "Our biological state is entwined with psychological, emotional, and spiritual health. This seems to add up to a different kind of healing, one that goes beyond cells and molecules to encompass our humanity too. . . . Researchers repeatedly find that people treated in a more holistic way do better physically as well as emotionally."[7]

Conventional medicine has its roots in cold, hard science. Underlying it is a concept called "materialism." The idea behind materialism in scientific study is that there is no such thing as an outcome being greater than the sum of its parts. All that exists is the matter we can objectively observe, and any activity, including consciousness, has its roots in physical matter. It's a great idea if scientists have to agree objectively on a study or theory. Materialism is important for the progression of scientific discovery and society at large because it excludes subjective opinions and beliefs. But individual patients have subjective experiences. Sometimes healing and human connection feel greater than the sum of their parts. Because science has a hard time pinning down things like love, belief, and perception, and pharmaceutical companies can't sell it in pill form—unless we include the placebo-equivalent effectiveness of some drugs—people are seeking an approach to medicine that includes this nonmaterialistic value system.

It doesn't mean they're engaging in quackery. Cannabis plants use their own cannabinoids to fight microbial and fungal pathogens[8] and protect them from UV light intensity.[9] Their sticky trichomes also reduce the stress of menacing insects, as spindly legs get stuck in the resin.[10] Thus, as the stress of their environment intensifies, they seem to benefit from producing more cannabinoids. When we ingest phytocannabinoids, they bond to our very cells. Some say cannabis eases stress, makes them feel alive in the present moment, or at one with nature. Scientifically, we may roll our eyes at such statements, but philosophically speaking, these are profound ideas. Plants can't run away or change their environment. Have they evolved the ability to *feel* okay about where they are? What is the consciousness of a plant, and since we share a common ancestor, can we access their consciousness?

I have no scientific study to back up my hypothesis, but is it possible that the endocannabinoid system is the point at which plant consciousness and human consciousness meet? Perhaps consciousness is a spectrum with plants on one end and us at the other. We can't observe it through a microscope, but we can observe its effects and should address it with science, just as we do dark matter, which makes up over 90 percent of the mass of the universe—despite our inability to observe it directly.[11] Applying science to consciousness is slippery, but I believe that the universe we inhabit within our own minds is more than just the sum of its observable parts. A study by the neuroscientist Dr. Sam Harris concluded that expression of beliefs, whether religious or verifiable facts, lit up the same part of the brain.[12] So it behooves us to acknowledge the gray area of consciousness and belief when we are treating sick people. If we are talking about medicine that alters consciousness, and consciousness does not require a definitive line between fact and fiction, then a response to a medicine like cannabis will be more than the sum of its observable parts. This is territory the FDA cannot possibly cover in its rules for approving drugs. But we as practitioners and caretakers have the capacity to connect these seemingly unrelated dots when it comes to helping others—and in so doing, ensure moderate use. Using cannabis does not automatically equal drug abuse, just as having a glass of wine at dinner does not equal alcoholism.

If the rules of a debate are subjective, then one need not be a scientist or legal expert to win the perception debate. It is perception, after all, that is changing cannabis laws in states across the United States. Despite lack of FDA evidence, doctors see improvements in their patients. Caregivers and patients recognize relief of the symptom when they try properly formulated cannabis remedies. Some people are abusing the drug, their minds stuck in a synaptic rut of lethargy and apathy (or worse, anxiety and depression), but through education we can change the perception of cannabis from both sides of the debate. It requires more than scientific fact, knowledge of the justice system, or a medical degree. When it comes to framing reality without following objective rules, art school and learning to empathize with my patients thanks to my decade teaching high school dropouts have been ideal training.

Turning Over a New Leaf

If you're like me, after years of research, practice, and perseverance, your lush garden is flowing in the breeze, and your remedies are brewing in Crock-Pots, ready to be bottled up and given to ailing patients in your community; this is when the police come. If you are lucky, they'll just be responding to an erroneous 911 call and won't summon you to court, while they threaten to take away your children. In Massachusetts, I can now give my remedies away. I just can't sell them. Regardless of the law, my advice is to be as polite to law enforcement officers as possible. I still see on a regular basis the policemen who raided my home. (Recently I passed one in the grocery store, but alas, I couldn't get him to look me in the eye.) I'm glad I presented myself during the raid as upstanding and polite: a professional just running his business within the city's regulatory framework for home-based businesses.[13] I wasn't ashamed of what I had done, and I didn't hate the police for doing their job. They too live within my community and want to keep it safe from drug-addled criminals. It is a point we can both agree on.

Cannabis has many drug-addled users, but many in the cannabis underground and those who support it are not criminals, and they don't abuse drugs. They are good people, and they know someone who has benefited from a properly formulated cannabis remedy. They know that despite the law, adults should have access to that remedy—even if it is from a friend or neighbor. When law enforcement came to my door on that bright September day, I believed I was providing a benefit, but the community—and the judge—had the final say.

For months after the raid, I was in an existential crisis. I was out of a job, I was publicly known as a busted pot grower, and I had no leads on employers who wanted to hire the "marijuana guy," despite my compassion for ailing patients. I still had to pick up my kids from school and attend the PTO fundraisers. I could feel parents' eyes on me, and I wondered—on which side of the cannabis debate did they fall? Did they perceive me as a menace to their children or as a brave citizen fighting against outdated laws to help sick people? Mostly, parents congratulated me and told me to "keep fighting the good fight." Regardless of how I was perceived in the community, I still needed to pick up the pieces and find a source of legal income.

Paradoxically, although it had been nearly three years since the medical marijuana law passed, the one dispensary in Massachusetts approved for operation finally opened in my town, a week after I was raided. Its ranks were already full of cashiers who made a retail wage weighing out cannabis for the medical marijuana patients who lined up behind the counter. The patients who had medical marijuana ID cards did not have to show medical records to their doctors or be interviewed at the dispensary to determine their medical need. The retail clerks couldn't advise them medically, as the FDA had not determined any medical benefits to cannabis. Clerks did not get to observe the plants growing off-site in a massive warehouse and did not formulate custom remedies as I had. My expertise would be useless there, and I couldn't live on a retail wage. Plus, with the state's strict background checks for all dispensary employees, they were not about to risk hiring me in their first month of operation.

On one hand, I felt ashamed that I had chosen to grow cannabis, formulate remedies, and help patients on my own, instead of plodding through the proper channels to work at a dispensary. But on the other hand, I never wanted to work for a heavily guarded dispensary, serving a clientele I hadn't personally selected. I had helped so many people precisely because I did grow, collect data on, and formulate my own remedies. I got to sit down with caretakers and family members to learn their whole story and help them holistically. Unlike the dispensary, I didn't sell sugary edibles. And if I had been selling weed to random people who lined up to purchase it, wouldn't I be contributing to the possibility that cannabis might be getting into the wrong hands? I have heard several stories of customers buying cannabis legally at dispensaries in order to distribute it illegally to others. I am not arguing that dispensaries are unsafe, but the purported safety regulations dispensaries have to follow do not prevent diversion of marijuana.

I also began to feel that my small-scale, traditional approach to cannabis was appropriate, because everywhere I went for several months after the raid, I was applauded for my efforts, even in the most unlikely places. One afternoon I stopped at the pharmacy to pick up medication. Having succumbed to the laws and conventions of the modern world, I had begun taking a generic SSRI antidepressant to manage my stress and anxiety. I was no longer using any cannabis, as it was what had gotten me into trouble. Its stress-relieving effects had become anxiety inducing after the raid brought fear and uncertainty to my family. I had lost faith in it and turned to doctor-prescribed pharmaceuticals. As the pharmacist looked my name up on the computer, she reached her hand across the counter and patted my arm.

"I just want to let you know that I really think what you did was a good thing. You were helping a lot of people," she said. Perhaps she empathized with why I was now taking an antidepressant. She gave me the bottle of pills, and I guilelessly thanked her for her support. The last place I expected to get vocal support for my illegal drug activity was from the pharmacist, but it made sense. A lot of my clients used that pharmacy, and she also knew their struggles with symptoms and the side effects of powerful medications.

A few weeks after the raid, I went to the local high school to vote, and again, when a white-haired woman looked up my name, she stopped me before handing me a ballot. "Hey, I know who you are. I read about you in the paper. Thank you for your work in the community. We need more people like you."

I was still in shock from a public shaming and the career-stopping raid, but apparently there were people who considered my work important and even heroic. Cashiers at the grocery store, teachers in my kids' school, and neighbors all approached me to offer support and commend me for my efforts. Some knew the clients I had served. Others had followed my story in the newspaper, as editorial boards feared I might be a danger to the community, and community members voiced their outrage at the injustice of my prosecution. As my community voted by a 5-to-4 margin to support the medical marijuana measure, support came from the unlikeliest of places. My wife, reeling from the public shaming, was surprised to receive support at the insurance company when she went in to renew our homeowner's insurance. "It's just such a shame what they're doing to your husband. I know my mother would have died in a lot more pain if she hadn't had access to *it* at the end. God rest her soul," the adjuster remarked. It seemed I represented a view that few in the community felt safe enough to voice themselves. But I still hadn't had my day in court. My legal status was unpredictable.

The lawyers that helped me were my friends, they were passionate about justice, and they knew the protocol. I was told to start gathering letters of support from the patients I served. Support began to pour in from patients, friends, family, and community members. In private sessions with the prosecutor and my lawyer, I brought in patients such as Phyllis with the hip pain and David's widow Wendy, who shared how I helped them at a time when they were vulnerable. With this support from my community and patients pleading with the district attorney to leave me alone, the prosecutor and my lawyer eventually settled on an arrangement. Sufficient evidence was found to convict me of a serious crime, but my actions were deemed humanitarian. It was clear that I was serving sick people in the community. Its citizens thought it was a poor use of tax dollars to put someone like me behind bars. I would still have a court date at which the judge would either support or deny the outcome, but the agreement was that I would have three months of unsupervised probation and a clean record. If I won, I would set a new legal precedent in the state for distribution of a Schedule I substance on that scale.

I was truly terrified by the justice system and the power it had over me. But I brought my same honesty and empathy to my hours of testimony with the prosecutor as I did to my patients. I never believed that the outcome of my case would result in my spending time behind bars, because the facts, presented clearly by lucid and thoughtful individuals such as myself, my attorney, and my patients, were too clear to ignore. This illegal plant had nuance. Sentencing for cannabis distribution, especially in a state that had legalized its medical use, was no longer a black-and-white issue for state attorneys and law enforcement. After the prosecutor miraculously read the forty-plus letters from patients and their families that I provided, I asked him what he personally thought about all my client stories. He was an otherwise straight-and-narrow prosecutor who played fair but kept his own opinions close to the vest. I liked him because he reminded me of my most skeptical clients. He wasn't going to make any judgment until he knew all the facts and every angle to the story.

"You know, when medical marijuana passed, I assumed it was a hoax. I thought guys would just say their back hurt so they could get a marijuana card to smoke pot. But my opinions on the subject have changed. I can tell these patients have been helped. Medical marijuana is real. Plus, I've never really had the opportunity to have an in-depth and thoughtful discussion about the subject with a defendant." I thanked him for his honesty and didn't see him again until the court date.

A few days after speaking to the prosecutor, I was notified by the Department of Children and Families (DCF) that my case of parental neglect had been dropped. My children would not be interviewed by a case worker. The family lawyer I had asked to be present at the interview was in disbelief. In his twenty years of working with child neglect cases, he had never heard of a case being dropped without the children being interviewed. My community was a small one. I do not know what conversations occurred behind the closed doors of the DCF, but perhaps in light of the outpouring of community support, taking my children away would not be seen as politically appropriate. As of this writing, it is legal for adults over twenty-one in Massachusetts to cultivate cannabis and be in possession of limited quantities of marijuana. They can legally give an ounce away to a friend, but it is still considered parental neglect under federal law to have children in a home where a Schedule I substance is distributed. State workers are still mandated to submit a 51A form if cannabis is thought to be in the home of a parent. Until federal law changes, state legislatures still have work to do to protect law-abiding families. Towns passing moratoriums on the production or sale of legal marijuana within their city limits appear to be in denial of the fact that it is already legally allowed in every home in which children reside. Education is the better approach.

On the day of my arraignment in court, I got up and made breakfast for my family, as I usually did. I sat uncomfortably in my suit, eating oatmeal, while I chatted with my kids. They wanted to come to court with me, but we decided against it. My wife and I didn't want to appear exploitive by parading our well-adjusted children in front of the judge. If the judge applied the full extent of the law in my case, would we want our children watching as their father was sentenced to federal prison time?

I had never been in the courtroom before. I sat quietly next to my lawyer as we watched a few defendants stand up and speak to the judge with their public defenders. The courtroom was full of people, some of whom I recognized as my clients and their families. When I stood and the facts of my case were presented to the judge, I was brought back to the day of the raid. The prosecutor began in a monotone: "The raid on his home yielded sixty-seven marijuana plants, twenty one-gallon bags of marijuana, and fifty-nine jars of hash oil." Even as I stood there, the amounts sounded substantial. But "facts" in a marijuana case are up for a wide interpretation. Of those sixty-seven plants, close to half were tiny clones rooted to preserve my precious medical strains. The twenty gallon bags of marijuana were not THC-laden flower buds. They were bags of the same fresh leaves I gave to David and Wendy for his nightly anointing. The fifty-nine jars of "hash oil" were oils, tinctures, and CBD products all grouped together under the term "hash oil" because the police—despite my midraid tutelage—didn't know the difference. Only three of the jars contained actual hash oil that I was saving for my client with a particularly painful cancer on his face. He applied it topically, and it took away the pain.

The judge was brief. He could have applied the full extent of the law, but instead he remarked that he thought the three-month probation was a fair and reasonable conclusion to my case and struck his gavel. "Good luck," he smiled. Later I wondered if he knew some of my clients, too. Relieved by his ruling, I thanked him and turned to leave the courtroom. As I walked down the aisle, every person sitting on the packed benches stood and followed me out the door. I had no idea they were all there to hear the outcome of my case. I was reticent to be the voice of informed reason when it came to cannabis in my community, but I accepted the role.

But I assumed that role was over. For several months, I searched for and applied to jobs throughout my community. I felt so inspired by my work helping sick people with cannabis that I wanted another job where I could help people directly. I was not called in for a single interview. If the human resources people hadn't heard about me already, a simple Internet search of my name would reveal the headline, "Local Man Pleads Guilty in Drug Case." It did not say, "Local Man Potentially Extends Life of Terminal Cancer Patient," or, "Local Man Discovers Remarkable Medical Efficacy of Illicit Plant." To reporters with deadlines, I was just another guy caught selling weed. At a press conference after the court hearing, a reporter who showed up at my home the day of the raid, and who wrote about the case, asked me sarcastically, "What do you do for a living?" I lamely explained that I was a cannabis consultant and I helped patients understand how to properly use medicinal cannabis. Later, I regretted not asking why it hadn't occurred to him to read a more eloquent answer to that question on my public Web site.

Despite my wounded ego, calls began to trickle in. "Hi, my name is Helen. I heard about the trouble you were in, but my husband isn't able to find good advice from the dispensary or his doctor about medical marijuana, and we need your help. Are you still seeing clients?" Other calls came in from growers in my state who had gotten busted as well. They were family men with kids who grew pot in their basements to supplement their income and helped the sick people they knew. They wanted my advice on how to proceed. I put them in touch with my lawyers and supported them any way I could.

I realized that the education gap between the cannabis-consuming crowd, the powers that be, and the people in the community who could benefit from it was still wide. I had always sought to bridge that gap. I resumed consultations for clients, and they would lay out the various remedies they had purchased at the dispensary, scratching their heads. I taught octogenarian war veterans how to smoke marijuana, and I guided patients in making their own remedies from the dispensary cannabis they purchased. My particular formulations and strains of oils, tinctures, and other remedies were not available at the dispensary. None of my specific CBD products were available, either. I began to work with more and more patients in using my legal CBD formulations to reduce pain and anxiety, insomnia, and issues of the gut, among other ailments.

In the process of using CBD exclusively for my clients, and owing to the fact that I had stopped using THC myself for several months, I experimented more in using CBD on myself. Needing clarity of purpose to ascend from the postraid plateau that I found myself on, I didn't want to risk inducing anxiety with THC. But the SSRI that I was on had been unable to keep my anxiety at bay. After I increased my SSRI dosage, a seemingly paradoxical effect began to emerge. The longer I took it, the more frequently I seemed to wake up in a cold sweat, my limbs coursing with tension and nervous energy. I began to experiment with CBD at higher doses to combat it and discovered that I had been using too little. I recalculated my formulas and made them more concentrated. With a daily maintenance of 50 mg of CBD-infused olive oil taken before bed, my anxiety dropped significantly and I tapered off the SSRI, restoring my nervous system to balance. My faith in medical cannabis was renewed, as I felt the subtle benefits of cannabidiol working its magic. Along with other adults, I also began helping pet owners address their pets' anxiety, pain, and ailments. They too suffer, and many pets don't do well on pharmaceuticals.

Where Do We Go from Here?

It is difficult to touch on all the aspects of a single plant that is legal in some states, illegal in others, used recreationally for escape, recommended medically by doctors, or farmed for the production of utilitarian items such as rope or fabric. The industry is large enough and the science is evolving so rapidly that informed experts are needed at all levels. Most people agree that the relaxing of laws is inevitable, albeit plodding, as legislatures wring their hands about how to prevent diversion of the drug to kids. It is as if their own youthful experiments with marijuana led to a public catastrophe worse than the opioid epidemic, alcohol addiction, or a drug arrest record. But the industry is growing quickly. As of 2017, at roughly two hundred thousand and counting, there are approximately as many legal employees in the cannabis industry as there are physicians nationwide.[14] These employees serve over 1.5 million registered marijuana patients (nearly two-thirds of them are in California).[15] Many of these cannabis businesses still have trouble gaining access to traditional banking, owing to the reluctance of banks to accept deposits of money earned from a federally controlled substance. I assume that traditional banks have no problem providing services to companies that manufacture or sell opioids.

The District of Columbia and the thirty states that have marijuana laws on the books all have different sets of regulations. I will not go into all of the differences, but in light of the ease with which a homeowner can start producing his or her own medicinal marijuana, some of the regulations are perplexing. For example, in Alaska patients can cultivate up to six marijuana plants but are allowed to be in possession of only a single ounce of usable marijuana. My guess is that at harvest time, many of the legal growers are breaking the one-ounce limit, increasing their likelihood of (and anxiety over) prosecution. In Arkansas, where cultivation is not permitted, patients are allowed to possess 2.5 ounces. Unfortunately, although the state passed the law in 2016, no patients in Arkansas will be registered until 2018, when dispensaries are expected to open. I would imagine that terminally ill patients and their families are already breaking the law to acquire their 2.5 ounces. In California, possession of 8 ounces is allowed. In Colorado, anything over an ounce will get you busted. In Florida, only nonsmokable forms of THC are allowed. Thousands of miles away, in Hawaii, caregivers—although they are currently allowed to grow for patients—will, when dispensaries open in 2019, be prohibited from doing so. Limiting adults who can provide or grow unique strains of cannabis limits options for patients and turns gardeners into criminals.

As laws evolve from allowing medical marijuana only to legalizing cannabis for all adults, presumably these laws will become more reasonable. But few provide any regulations or standards for education, patient care, or medical expertise of industry employees. One helpful factor in almost every state is the requirement that all marijuana be tested for active cannabinoids, making it doubtful that we will return to the early 1900s, when few could distinguish between hemp and hash. Testing laboratories are a large component of many medical marijuana laws, yet access to technology to test cannabis is now available, making restrictions on home growers who can produce dispensary-grade cannabis unnecessary. If their products are free of contaminants, there is no difference between their products and that of a dispensary. Although dangerous molds can be found in any cannabis and do pose a health risk for patients with compromised immune systems,[16] the fear of contaminated cannabis can be overblown and misleading to consumers. Just as it is difficult to test the safety of every piece of meat sold in a supermarket, one part of a cannabis plant may be free of mold and another, an untested flower top, may contain it. In Massachusetts, strict regulations to avoid heavy-metal contaminants in cannabis are mandated, yet similar levels of analysis for alcohol, food, or other consumables are not required. When I corresponded with a commercial grower in the state who was prevented by the Department of Public Health from selling his dispensary's first crop of organically grown cannabis, owing to "high cadmium levels," he pointed out that a testing lab had found higher levels of cadmium in an organic potato procured at Whole Foods Market.[17]

Some entire countries are evolving in their marijuana laws, as well. Uruguay, the first country to legalize the drug in 2013, has yet to succumb to reefer madness. Although the industry will be state run, the "great experiment," as it has been dubbed, seems reasonable. Home cultivation will be allowed, and clubs or associations will be able to grow cannabis for members. The taxes from sales will then support addiction and youth drug prevention, as well as other social services. The taxes will be low at first, since the government plans to sell a gram of cannabis for $1.30, less than a tenth of the average gram price in America.[18] Alas, sales to foreign tourists will be illegal. Who wants tourists from all over the world flooding Uruguay with their money? Colorado alone has generated billions of dollars of tax revenue since legalization.

Canada is also moving forward with a full legalization effort. The Canadian system is not perfect, but currently, caregivers selling medical marijuana can set up online businesses. This is a reasonable response to the fear of untoward pot shops cluttering up shopping districts with neon pot signs. Still, the proposed legalization falls short of truly addressing the youth issue. As if the state will have any control over a product's ultimate ingestion by an individual, it maintains a commitment to "tracking of cannabis from seed to sale to prevent diversion to the illicit market."[19] Some health professionals are recommending that the minimum age to buy legal marijuana be set at twenty-five years of age. This seems reasonable for protecting the healthy developing brain, even if the verdict is out on whether the brain is negatively affected. But it does little to help young people like Heather in chapter 4 who have a terminal disease and could benefit from marijuana. The 2018 law will allow all adults over eighteen to buy pot, but the irony is that a caregiver like me (or a parent) who provides cannabis oil to a child like Heather will serve a jail sentence of up to fourteen years.[20] Israel, which has led the clinical research on medical cannabis for decades, has a system that is both rational and conservative. Although it is not legal for adult use, state-regulated cannabis producers create products for the country's more than twenty-five thousand medical marijuana patients, and researchers are allowed to perform controlled trials on the drug's efficacy.[21]

The round peg of marijuana may never fully fit into the square hole of regulations. Despite the U.S. marijuana industry generating close to $7 billion worth of revenue in 2016,[22] in 2010, the last year data were available, the federal government was still spending $17 billion a year fighting production and distribution of the plant.[23] The number of tax dollars spent on law enforcement for possession in legal states will inevitably go down. But there is another economic burden one could add to the billions of dollars Americans spend to fight marijuana: the cost of the opioid epidemic. At over $78 billion a year in the United States,[24] the price society pays to fight opioid overdose, abuse, and dependence compounds the economic burden and irony of fighting cannabis, an herbal drug that has been proven to reduce opioid use in states where it is legal. (It reduces opioids in other states too. People are just hiding their use.) The findings from a study conducted by the National Bureau of Economic Research are sobering. The study revealed that

> states with licensed Marijuana Dispensaries (LMDs) had lower opioid-overdose mortality rates and fewer admissions to treatment for opioid addiction than they would have had without the dispensaries. The estimated sizes of the reductions were 16 to 31 percent in mortality due to prescription opioid overdoses, and 28 to 35 percent in admissions for treatment of opioid addiction. This latter reduction was steeper, up to 53 percent, among patients who entered treatment independently of the criminal justice system. The researchers also noted a trend whereby the longer LMDs were in place, the more the incidence of opioid-related problems declined.[25]

If my pain clients are any indication, then more cannabis dispensaries, consultants, and householders alike are needed to fight another drug war: the war to reduce harmful pharmaceuticals. I do worry about the effect chronic cannabis use has on children's developing brains. But that level of worry is akin to wondering if too much screen time is affecting their brains. Whether pot or screens are harmful, the danger of opioid addiction and overdose represents another level of worry for parents that is more significant.

When it is helping pain sufferers taper off their opioids or autistic teens stay focused in school, cannabis done correctly is another option that can bring health and renewal to the sick where many drugs fail. At times, marijuana's use in society becomes out of balance, just like our health and our health care system. High THC strains can dominate the field, and many people succumb to its addictive, mind-fogging, or anxiety-inducing effects. Used unchecked, it becomes a drug of escape and recreation. But the majority of Americans are aware that despite these pitfalls, the time to fight it is over. A nationwide poll in 2014 found that *90 percent* of Americans supported legalizing medical marijuana.[26] This brings us to an interesting crossroads in marijuana's history in the United States. With 90 percent of Americans supporting legalization, and 13 percent of medical schools studying its effect on the endocannabinoid system, we may enter an era where cannabis is akin to alcohol: sold to adults from stores without the holistic education that should go hand in hand with using the drug properly.

I am not conservative when it comes to marijuana laws. On the contrary: I support complete and total legalization of marijuana for adults (and medical access for children). I believe in relaxing all irrational laws that claim to regulate it. It is thriving already and will continue to exist in black and white markets at every level of consumption, from neighbors exchanging remedies to established dispensaries like Harborside in Oakland, California, which serves over two hundred thousand registered patients.[27] Most marijuana laws could effectively fit within the current regulations governing liquor stores, breweries, wineries, saloons, and coffee shops.

Although many of the data show that teen marijuana use,[28] driving fatalities,[29] and crime[30] do not increase in states that have legalized marijuana, I based my legalization opinion on the pharmaceutical and chemical context cannabis resides within. The number of FDA-approved drugs taken off the market for the harms they later were found to have caused is in the dozens.[31] Without a single fatality caused by cannabis in its 4,500 years of written history, fearing the unknown harms of cannabis is a laughable and amoral excuse for not approving it as a drug with medical benefits. The many drugs later pulled from the market (let alone the dangerous drugs still on the market) are proof that the FDA has a long history of approving drugs that have killed, maimed, or driven users to kill others. Vioxx, a drug linked to over twenty-seven thousand heart attacks,[32] is a good case in point. Recent data collected on the effects of cannabidiol (CBD) show it to be comparable in its ability to reduce inflammation to Vioxx, which was pulled off the market in 2004 after being prescribed to twenty million people.[33]

Add to this the tens of thousands of chemicals in shampoos, soaps, food production, cosmetics, and industrial applications. Only a small fraction of them have been deemed safe by the Environmental Protection Agency, which regulates their safety.[34] The FDA is not mandated to test whether these thousands of chemicals that go into our bodies and our children's are safe.

My liberal views on legalization do not mean that I support the often low-consciousness or stereotypical culture that goes along with the drug. In that regard, I am conservative. Just as Ralph Nader's critique of the auto industry—*Unsafe at Any Speed*—helped change the culture of vehicle production from no safety standards to car companies competing with one another in the number of safety features they offered, I believe that the culture and knowledge around cannabis can and must change if we are to derive a benefit for our communities. Providing education and safety to consumers and communities is a productive way for dispensaries to compete for and attract new clientele.

My views on legalization are not unique. They are articulated well by the Unitarian Universalist Association (commonly known as the Unitarian Church), which has supported drug legalization since 1970. Their strategy is commendable because it takes into account the holistic approach needed to keep communities safe. Although I am quoting a large section, it is an important reminder of the commitment required to keep kids safe. This is from their "Statement of Conscience" concerning the war on drugs:

> We must begin with ourselves. Our congregations can offer safe space for open and honest discussion among congregants about the complex issues of drug use, abuse, and addiction. Through acceptance of one another and the encouragement of spiritual growth, we should be able to acknowledge and address our own drug use without fear of censure or reprisal.
>
> We can recognize that drugs include not only currently illegal substances but also alcohol, nicotine, caffeine, over-the-counter pain relievers, and prescription drugs. We can learn to distinguish among use, abuse, and addiction. We can support one another in recognizing drug-related problems and seeking help. We can seek to understand those among us who use drugs for relief or escape. With compassion, we can cultivate reflection and analysis of drug policy. In the safe space of our own congregations, we can begin to prevent destructive relationships with drugs. We can lend necessary support to individuals and families when their loved ones need treatment for addiction problems. We can encourage our congregations to partner with and follow the lead of groups representing individuals whose lives are most severely undermined by current drug policy—people of color and people of low income. We can learn from health care professionals what the unique patterns of substance abuse are in our local areas. We can go beyond our walls and bring our perspective to the interfaith community, other nonprofit organizations, and elected officials.[35]

This process is beginning in the industry, and many of the industry's early advocates subscribe to a conservative approach to marijuana. The National Organization for the Reform of Marijuana Laws developed the *Principles of Responsible Use,* which focuses on appropriate adult consumption, responsible driving, proper setting, respecting the rights of others, and resisting abuse.[36] Cannabis cultivators are also bringing the more subtle cannabinoids like CBD back into balance and are creating strains that reflect our need for stability and health without the "high." Cannabis schools and training organizations have been established that seek to educate bud tenders and industry workers. Bringing cannabis into the light and into the hands of law-abiding citizens will also help this evolution, but the culture of intimacy, empathy, and healing that has evolved along with home cannabis cultivation can coincide with and influence the industry if it is allowed to. Cannabis schools can and will educate students about the scientific and social complexities of cannabis, but I still believe a person with years of experience in growing, formulating remedies, and treating patients firsthand, with the strains he or she knows intimately, will be a more successful and empathic practitioner than someone who has never touched the plant. These practitioners are already out there, hiding in the shadows. Their expertise is needed in nursing homes, hospitals, and at hospice facilities. They are needed in educating health practitioners, legislatures, and citizens. Their expertise is crucial in winning *both* the drug wars. They should not be forced deeper into the underground by regulations that encourage only "big marijuana" to survive. If my business had not been raided, my earnings would have easily broken six figures. Few home growers will be incentivized to work for a retail wage at a dispensary or cultivation site. As prices fall and legal access to marijuana increases, their basement businesses will fade away, their unique medicinal strains and knowledge fading out as well. I hope my story shows that we should not accept this loss because we believe that regulated dispensaries are protecting children better than the homeowners who live in and interact with their communities.

As I did with the prosecutor in my legal case, regulations and communities might encourage dispensaries to provide evidence that they are reducing symptoms, increasing quality of life, and decreasing the use of harmful medication by their patients. These data can be collected anonymously via software from the moment a patient enters a dispensary. Where dispensaries are failing to sustain a net benefit to their customers, cannabis experts who understand the process from *seed to cell* can help hone a dispensary's processing, delivery, and education system. In the future, dispensaries that can prove they are providing the highest net benefit to their community will be sought after.

Dispensary software can also easily address the issue of chronic use and overdose by having grading systems for new or experienced users. New users will be started on mild products, and experienced users will have access to stronger concentrations. Software can alert bud tenders to check in with patients who might be purchasing an inordinate amount or when an anxiety sufferer is using a strain that others have reported only increased their anxiety. Software can also address an issue in legal marijuana states with what's called "loopers." These are customers who come from out of state to buy the maximum daily amount of cannabis legally at a dispensary, in order to then sell it in states where it is illegal. It is the definition of diversion and might happen less at community-oriented, small-scale dispensaries that know their customers. Software could catch much of this activity, quelling the fears of states that are bordering legal states (but that haven't done their research into the benefits of legalization). But the responsibility does not rest entirely with the dispensary. Legislatures, community leaders, and citizens need to engage with experts in the industry, as well as the people who use cannabis, in order to best understand the movement of the drug, legal or not. Controlling diversion requires more than the stroke of the governor's pen.

Laws cannot mandate empathic approaches to legal cannabis, but the best way for a dispensary to provide a sustainable service to the town it resides within is to demonstrate to the community that it has the best interests of patients, parents, police, and everyone else involved at heart. I do believe there is room for large-scale dispensaries, ma-and-pa shops, and law-abiding home cultivators, but just because a dispensary has the capital to jump through every regulatory hoop does not mean that every client is safely using its product. In states where only uninformed bureaucracy, tax revenue, and investor profits are driving the industry, experienced cannabis householders have a role. I encourage them to advertise their services as compassionate, informed cannabis consultants who can provide a link between dispensaries, consumers, health organizations, and the community at large. Reach out to doctors, health practitioners, and dispensaries with your educational services.

Health providers will send patients to the professionals in the community who are informed and have health in mind. And for every person who is comfortable waiting in a dispensary line to buy marijuana, there are others who would prefer a private transaction with a neighbor or practitioner they know and trust. As they have for decades, cannabis householders should also be legally allowed to derive income from serving these people. To my mind, a masseuse, an acupuncturist, an Ayurvedic practitioner, or a chiropractor should be allowed to sell cannabis products to her clients or use them in treatments. Do we think a chiropractor is more likely to divert marijuana to children, or a for-profit dispensary that serves hundreds of thousands of customers? Would you more readily trust your masseuse or a glassy-eyed bud tender half your age for guidance on using a topical cannabis for muscle pain? Marijuana laws should allow for individuals who already have medical practices and cannabis expertise to advise and sell cannabis to their patients. This is the safest way to prevent the diversion of marijuana, because these professionals are committed health practitioners who want to keep their standing in the community. If we truly care about the health of our communities, then we will allow those who already heal to heal with cannabis.

Recontextualizing Cannabis

Pot smokers and growers who grow cannabis to escape from reality should not be in jail, in my opinion. But many are ashamed of their pot use, even if it is helping them medically. If we as cannabis consumers are hyperparanoid of revealing our use, we are delaying the progression of reform. If we neither learn the facts nor share our knowledge with sick people who could benefit from cannabis, and we do nothing for cannabis advocacy, then our communities will not benefit. People will overdose on opioids. Children will suffer in hospitals with their terminal diseases, their bodies loaded up on pharmaceuticals, their parents heartbroken.

Likewise, if cannabis professionals do not elevate the dialogue on medical marijuana, legislatures will not regulate the industry to be patient focused, and big dispensaries churning out cannabis to heavy users will be the norm. The recreational market may overtake the medical marijuana market, leaving uninformed patients and those who could benefit from holistic, traditionally formulated cannabis behind. If we remain silent, we are undermining those who are more vocal about the cause but are still being persecuted. We are perpetuating the stereotypes of cannabis being an illicit drug that one should feel guilty using.

Cannabis users have reason to be fearful of law enforcement, but if you're a cannabis householder and otherwise law-abiding citizen, then your community could benefit from your story. There is a difference between breaking the law and breaking one's ethical or moral code. Cannabis laws are wrong because they are based on cultural perception, not science and facts. Breaking irrational cannabis laws is a form of civil disobedience that protests injustice. We allow drug manufacturers to advertise dangerous drugs on television, despite the overdose epidemic ravaging this country. Our culture does not perceive this as wrong. Meanwhile, adults can be sentenced to decades in prison for selling a joint to a friend.[37] In many countries, their fate can be worse. If you believe your legal or illegal use of cannabis can be supported ethically, then write an anonymous letter to your local paper stating your role in the community and your healthy use of cannabis. Tell your doctors about it, and take them to task if they don't know the science behind cannabinoids, both endo- and phyto-. Your doctors are legally bound to keep your medical information private. When I hear clients say that their doctors dismiss any medical claims for cannabis, I suggest they ask their doctors to show objective proof. I also suggest they ask their doctor to show them the evidence of a prescribed drug's safety by comparison with cannabis. Anyone who types the name of a drug and "side effects" or "fatalities" into a search engine should have enough information to start the conversation with his or her doctor.

If you hide your cannabis use out of shame or because you subconsciously believe you are a druggie, then are you? What is driving your shame? If you are thoughtlessly consuming marijuana with no medicinal frame of reference, then I believe you are doing little for the cannabis movement and little for patients who could desperately use the medicine you consume. You have a right to keep your cannabis use private, but your views on it should be shared—because most likely, you're *not* a druggie. Chances are, your marijuana use helps you sleep, takes the edge off your stressful job, or keeps your menstrual cramps and aches and pains at bay. Your doctor or pharmacist could benefit from hearing about cannabis from a nice person like you who isn't smoking a joint in public or donning a pot leaf cap.

For those cannabis-friendly citizens out there who do proudly don the pot leaf cap, clearly you are not afraid of being out of the cannabis closet. If so, there is more you can do to help the cause. Aside from learning the science and history behind cannabis, there are facets of cannabis activism that are easy to get involved in but rarely explored. Social media apps are full of videos depicting people consuming the plant or growing it in undisclosed locations, but rarely do we see this plant freed from the heavily guarded dispensary grows, basements, and secret mountain glens where it is produced. The living cannabis plant is marijuana in its purest and most benign form. Because the drug war has inflated the price of this roadside weed, we think it is too valuable a commodity to waste by planting it in a public place as a political statement. But I believe the plant needs to be set free to help elevate the conversation. You can easily take the seeds you find in your cannabis, or the extra rooted clones your friends have in their grow spaces, and plant them outside in the summer. Place them in flower pots on boulevards, in the gardens surrounding the governor's mansion, or in the window boxes in front of the police station. The plants need to be alive only long enough to capture an image that is both shocking and banal: a cannabis plant in public, nestled among its more ostentatious (and often more toxic) flowering friends. One image of a cannabis plant growing in a police station flower box posted on social media would help remind the world of this drug's humble origins. Yes, it will be cut down immediately by the authorities. But the image will inspire people in other towns and other countries to begin a rational discussion on the topic. No, we're not trying to get kids hooked on pot. We're trying to get adults off the pills that have hooked them.

If guerrilla gardening is too extreme for your taste, you can help shift public perception in other ways. A campus quad gathering of twenty-somethings smoking pot sends a tired and outdated message: yes, twenty-somethings smoke pot. Instead, organize a public chess tournament with stoned participants, a "420" trivia night, or cannabis-infused athletic competition. Science majors can perform their own research trials on cannabis when they track wins by stoned or sober chess players, or perform double-blind tests on their friends to determine whether a strain or terpene profile is sativa or indica, anxiety-provoking or anxiety-reducing. The data collected may not be published on the National Institutes of Health Web site, but could sway some skeptical parents and professors. Elevating the dialogue on cannabis would help send an updated message: yes, productive, intellectually engaged citizens smoke pot. Certainly, Cannabis Cup competitions, which showcase the fruits of talented pot growers, can expand to include such events.

If you are connected with law enforcement or know someone who is, then you have a role to play as well. Ask yourself: "What is the safest net benefit to society—using enforcement resources to eradicate the ubiquitous backyard cannabis plant, or devoting them to saving lives in the opioid epidemic?" What is a better fulfillment of the police catchphrase, "to protect and serve"? Many police officers will wash their hands of the cannabis issue by saying they're just doing their job. But true justice comes to communities when all sides are informed and aware of the consequences of outdated laws that affect people unfairly. The DEA does not have absolute authority over the land. Even law enforcement officers can suggest to their superiors that objective, unbiased information be offered about cannabis and the laws that regulate it. The police officers who raided me had a genuine curiosity about the products brewing in my home. Perhaps a formal class on the difference between hash oil and CBD oil would streamline law enforcement resources. A handheld cannabinoid tester to determine this difference is an inexpensive investment for a police department. More in-depth discussions also need to take place between prosecutors and law enforcement, because families are still being torn apart by a plant that is now helping sick people in a majority of states.

Law Enforcement Action Partnership (LEAP), an organization run by retired law enforcement officers dedicated to ending cannabis prohibition, has a national platform for helping communities rethink and evolve their approach to prohibition and legalization. Police chiefs in cities where legal cannabis is regulated understand the pitfalls and benefits of legalization. They may not have time to speak to a cannabis consultant or parent of a teenager with juvenile Huntington's disease. But they can make time for fellow police chiefs who want the facts and want to stay in the good graces of the communities they protect.

Another major area of cannabis injustice yet to be reformed is workplace drug testing. Employers who still conduct drug tests of their employees and who care about the bottom line when it comes to workplace morality and productivity would do well to open up a dialogue about appropriate marijuana use among their employees, especially in states where it is legal for adults. The practice of drug testing and firing workers who have THC in their system, regardless of whether the THC was ingested days or weeks beforehand, is a waste of valuable resources. Money spent on drug testing for THC, which can linger in one's system for weeks after it is ingested, could be better spent on other employee programs, such as new skills training, team building, workplace efficiency, and safety (in addition to education about alcohol and opioid addiction). If you are an employer hiring adults and imposing drug testing in a state that has legalized the adult use of marijuana, you are depriving your business of valuable talent, promoting unemployment, and damaging the economy that will help your business grow. You are denying your company of good workers, on the basis of an irrational fear that somehow a joint smoked on Friday night will affect the productivity of a worker come Monday morning.

Legislatures also have to take a rational and informed stance when writing cannabis laws. The plant will inevitably be grown by green-thumbed citizens who *accidentally* end up with far more than they can reasonably consume or even give away. What then? My father lives in Colorado and was given a full-grown plant by a neighbor at harvest time. Although he didn't really want it, my father cured the half pound of potent cannabis and kept it stored in a dozen jars. He even made a wooden pipe to try a couple puffs but quickly determined his pot-smoking days were over. The marijuana was just too strong. Law prevents him from selling it legally, but why? What else can he do with it? If he had a proper laboratory analysis of his product, wouldn't it be more appropriate to let a dispensary dispense it to patients in need of potent medicine? Laws that prevent individual growers from selling their surplus to medical dispensaries *encourage* diversion of marijuana, in my opinion. Laws that allow people to "give away" marijuana without remuneration are also myopic. We live in a capitalist, market-driven society. Those who run legal businesses out of their own homes contribute openly to their local economy. Cannabis is a valuable medicine and cannabis householders should be allowed to profit from their labor as any other small farmers do.

Perhaps cannabis laws will eventually allow for farmer's markets and roadside cannabis stands where individuals can peddle their small yet prized harvests to those who show ID. My local farmer's market sells wine and provides tastings. Is it unreasonable to think that cannabis could also fit into the farmer's market tradition once we free our minds from the irrational fears and stereotypes we place upon it? I know a cannabis grower who happens to sell his legal salad greens at the local farmer's market. He's excited for the marijuana laws to evolve, not so he can sell weed from his booth. He wants to sell sprouted cannabis seedlings for salads. The laws should allow for this. What legal dispensary sells cannabis sprouts?

Those who are bold enough to enact these creative and harmless experiments in recontextualizing cannabis are often smeared across the media. A sprout seller may get the headline "Man Secretly Sells Pot at Farmer's Market," where "Man Pushes Boundaries of Outdated Cannabis Laws at Farmer's Market" would be a more appropriate choice. This is because reporters and the press also have a role to play in changing stereotypes. Often, articles detailing the scientific breakthroughs on cannabis research still use unscientific words like "pot" and "weed." Adderall is a drug that helps (and hinders) thousands of patients, but rarely do headlines touting its medicinal efficacy refer to it as *meth,* its slang term and identical molecular counterpart.[38] When citizens are arrested for cultivating or dispensing cannabis, reporters can do more research on the clientele and the products being sold. What was the cannabinoid content of the products? Are there patients with terminal or life-threatening diseases who are suddenly without a supply of a medicine? What is their story? Will the "drug dealer's" pain clients increase their opioid use when their pot supply is cut off? How does that affect the reporter's beat? By now, reporters have enough evidence at their fingertips to know that a cannabis drug bust may be hurting innocent people in the community as well. A local grower recently approached me, as he was inspired to share his story of how his daily use of large amounts of raw cannabis juice kept his epilepsy at bay. He cannot tolerate the psychoactive aspects of the plant, and after years of experimentation he found that the raw juice was more effective—but it required him to grow a substantial amount of cannabis. Several weeks after our conversation, I saw in the paper that he had been raided by police. The article mentioned only that law enforcement had found cannabis in excess of the legal limit, and his mug shot was printed alongside the article.

I experienced a grand mal seizure in my youth due to a head injury, and my heart aches at his predicament.

What about the institutions that are full of the very people who can most benefit from reducing symptoms and increasing quality of life? Shouldn't nursing homes and patient care facilities be allowed to grow resident-maintained cannabis gardens that help reduce the health care costs of the facility and boost healthy gardening activity? Certainly, senior citizens can be trusted to safely derive the euphoric, pain-relieving, and neuroprotective benefits of cannabis in their old age. Are we worried they might give it to their grandchildren on the side or become addicted? Again, the legal pills in their medicine cabinets are already fulfilling this role. Small institutions that provide care for elderly adults are an ideal setting for a knowledgeable grower to apply his or her skills. One skilled practitioner, with the help of geriatric volunteers, could provide cannabis remedies and guidance to the residents of the facility.

I know doctors are still wary of drugs without FDA approval. Perhaps they are worried about the stigma or the potential harms of cannabis. All attributes of cannabis need to be addressed more thoroughly and objectively by researchers. But doctors and health care providers hold the key, I believe, to allowing cannabis to truly benefit the infirm. Doctors need to look deep into their souls and ask themselves what a vow to "do no harm" means when they prescribe drugs that kill or maim. About one in three doctors is in the top 1 percent of the nation's wealthiest households in the country.[39] Such physicians have access to the health care that this wealth brings. It is ironic that some of the most privileged few are in charge of the care of those who suffer the most. People in privileged positions have to work harder to learn empathy. Hospitals and doctors' offices could reduce the pressure of too many patients and costly medical errors if they brought professional cannabis experts in to advise on the subject. In Massachusetts, where medical and adult-use marijuana is legal for everyone over twenty-one, most hospitals and doctors' offices have no clear policies about whether patients should medicate with the drug on site or be thrown out by the police. In their defense, the organizations may be subject to federal law because of funding, or they may not have the expertise to separate the abusive cannabis users from those who desperately need it to assuage their suffering. Hiring a cannabis consultant or training staff to understand appropriate medical marijuana use is a simple step. I have been encouraged to speak at hospitals, but I do not meet the requirement of having a medical degree. I had to publish a book to prove my cannabis knowledge.

There are others who could benefit from cannabis information and sensible laws. Currently, investment in the legal cannabis industry benefits those who have the money to invest, but I do think about the communities of color or areas in poverty that have borne the brunt of the drug war. Perhaps nuanced cannabis regulation could benefit communities, economically as well as medically, that have utilized it for generations. I envision rooftop cannabis gardens on urban apartment buildings run by tenants who dispense it to ailing community members. The cannabis is grown by and for the communities. It provides jobs, eases stress, and reduces public health care costs. Where addiction and misuse occur, the community and drug counselors, not the police, can intervene. Those who fall in love with the act of growing cannabis do not wish to see the fruits of their labor debilitate its consumers or drive them to darkness. Where profits (driven by inordinate taxation, fees, and regulation) are not the motivation, I believe that balance and health will occur.

There are far too many historical elements, practical uses, and scientific aspects of cannabis for one book to cover, but with a more informed, empathic, and medicinal stance on the drug, marijuana dispensaries and householders will better serve their communities. We don't know how long draconian laws will control this plant worldwide, but with reform, those who suffer will benefit. Those in jail will return to productive lives. Those with cannabis expertise will have a legal framework within which to share their knowledge. There is only one way to find out the extent to which we can all benefit from embracing this medicinal plant, and that is to try.

Notes

Introduction

1. O. H. G. Wilder-Smith and L. Arendt-Nielsen, "Postoperative Hyperalgesia: Its Clinical Importance and Relevance," *Anesthesiology* 104(3) (March 2006): 601–607.

ONE Confessions of a Cannabis Consultant

1. Arcview Market Research & BDS Analytics, *The State of Legal Marijuana Markets,* 5th ed., 2017, accessed October 31, 2017, www.arcviewmarketresearch.com.

2. Julie Holland, ed., *The Pot Book: A Complete Guide to Cannabis* (Rochester, VT: Park Street Press, 2010).

3. Hong-En Jiang, et al., "A New Insight into *Cannabis sativa* (Cannabaceae) Utilization from 2,500-Year-Old Yanghai Tombs, Xinjiang, China," *Journal of Ethnopharmacology* 108(3) (December 6, 2006): 414–422.

4. Ethan Russo, "Cannabis in India: Ancient Lore and Modern Medicine," in R. Mechoulam, ed., *Cannabinoids as Therapeutics,* 1–22 (Basel, Switzerland: Birkhäuser Verlag, 2005).

5. Prashanti de Jager, Holistic Academy lecture, Track I, Module 6: "The Ayurvedic + Vedic Constituents of Cannabis," 2017.

6. Russo, "Cannabis in India."

7. Natalya M. Kogan and Rapahel Mechoulam, "Cannabinoids in Health and Disease," *Dialogues in Clinical Neuroscience* 9(4) (2007): 413–430.

8. Wen Jiang et al., "Cannabinoids Promote Embryonic and Adult Hippocampus Neurogenesis and Produce Anxiolytic- and Antidepressant-like Effects," *Journal of Clinical Investigation* 115(11) (2005): 3104–3116.

9. Maureen Dowd, "Don't Harsh Our Mellow, Dude," *New York Times* op-ed column, June 3, 2014.

10. Ethan Russo, "History of Cannabis and Its Preparations in Saga, Science, and Sobriquet," *Chemistry and Biodiversity* 4 (2007): 1614–1648.

11. Ibid.

12. Ibid.

13. Holland, *The Pot Book.*

14. Ibid.

15. Ibid.

16. Robert Deitch, *Hemp—American History Revisited: The Plant with a Divided History* (New York: Algora Publishing, 2003), 16.

17. Dale H. Gieringer, "The Forgotten Origins of Cannabis Prohibition in California," *Contemporary Drug Problems, Federal Legal Publications, New York* 26(2) (summer 1999).

18. Anna Berkes, "Some of My Finest Hours Have Been Spent on My Back Veranda, Smoking Hemp," *Thomas Jefferson Encyclopedia,* "Spurious Quotations," July 23, 2010, www.monticello.org, accessed November 2, 2017.

19. Donald Jackson, ed., *The Diaries of George Washington* (Charlottesville: University Press of Virginia, 1976–1979), 1:340.

20. W. B. O'Shaughnessy, "On the Preparations of the Indian Hemp, or Gunjah (*Cannabis indica*): Their Effects on the Animal System in Health, and Their Utility in the Treatment of Tetanus and Other Convulsive Diseases," *Provincial Medical Journal and Retrospect of the Medical Sciences* 5(123) (1843): 363–369.

21. Baron Ernst von Bibra, *Plant Intoxicants: A Classic Text on the Use of Mind-Altering Plants,* translated by Hedwig Schleiffer (Rochester, VT: Healing Arts Press, 1995). Originally published 1855.

22. O'Shaughnessy, "On the Preparations of the Indian Hemp."

23. Russo, "Cannabis in India."

24. H. H. Kane, *Drugs That Enslave: The Opium, Morphine, Chloral and Hashisch Habits* (Philadelphia: Presley Blakiston, 1881), 207–208.

25. Dale Gieringer, "125th Anniversary of the First U.S. Anti-Drug Law: San Francisco's Opium Den Ordinance (Nov. 15, 1875)," DrugSense.org, November 2000, accessed October 31, 2017, http://www.drugsense.org/dpfca/opiumlaw.html.

26. Robert Connell Clark, *Hashish!* (Los Angeles: Red Eye Press, 1998) 223, 233.

27. "Section 3874, Revised Statutes, Missouri, 1889," *British Medical Journal* 1 (June 5, 1897): 1092.

28. "Haschisch Candy," *Boston Medical and Surgical Journal* 75 (November 22, 1866): 348–350.

29. Cited in Michael Aldrich, "A Brief Legal History of Marihuana" (Phoenix: Do It Now Foundation, 1971).

30. "Section 3874, Revised Statutes."

31. "It Brings Ravishing Dreams of Bliss," *San Francisco Call,* October 24, 1897, p. 17.

32. Gieringer, "The Forgotten Origins of Cannabis Prohibition in California."

33. Ibid.

34. "There are but few people in this State who know that 'hashish,' the opium of Arabs, is raised, prepared, smoked and eaten in California the same as along the eastern shores of the Mediterranean and Red seas. . . . Arabs and Armenians or Turks Are Growing Twenty Acres of Hemp Near Stockton," *San Francisco Call,* June 24, 1895.

35. Caleb Hellerman, "Scientists Say the Government's Only Pot Farm Has Moldy Samples—and No Federal Testing Standards," PBS News Hour, March 8, 2017, accessed October 31, 2017, http://www.pbs.org/newshour/updates/scientists-say-governments -pot-farm-moldy-samples-no-guidelines/.

36. It is interesting to note that although Anslinger is associated with many racist comments linking cannabis with minorities, tangible evidence for his actually making them is nonexistent.

37. Harry J. Anslinger and Will Oursler Farrar, *The Murderers: The Story of Narcotics Gangs* (New York: Straus and Cudahy, 1961).

38. Credited to John Ehrlichmann (1994). Ehrlichmann's family has denied the veracity of this statement. Quoted in article by Dan Baum, who "remembered" it from an interview twenty-two years earlier, "Legalize It All: How to Win the War on Drugs," *Harper's Magazine* (April 2016).

39. Sarah E. Boslaugh, *The SAGE Encyclopedia of Pharmacology and Society* (Thousand Oaks, CA: Sage, 2015), 1758.

40. J. D. House, J. Neufeld, and G. Leson, "Evaluating the Quality of Protein from Hemp Seed (*Cannabis sativa* L.) Products through the Use of the Protein Digestibility–Corrected Amino Acid Score Method," *Journal of Agricultural Food Chemistry* 58(22) (November 24, 2010): 11801–11807.

41. "California Proposition 215, the Medical Marijuana Initiative (1996)," BallotPedia at www.ballotpedia.org, accessed November 3, 2017.

42. Oregon Health Authority, Oregon Medical Marijuana Program, "Medical

Marijuana Rules and Statutes OAR 333–007: Marijuana Labeling and Concentration Limits, Effective May 31, 2017."

43. Ibid.

44. John M. McPartland, "The Endocannabinoid System: An Osteopathic Perspective," *Journal of the American Osteopathic Association* 108 (October 2008): 586–600.

45. David Allen et al., "A Survey of American Medical School's Acceptance of the Science of the ECS (Endocannabinoid System)," *Cannabisdigest.ca* (July 18, 2014), accessed October 31, 2017, https://cannabisdigest.ca/survey-endocannabinoid-system-medical-schools/.

46. Ibid.

47. Holland, *The Pot Book.*

48. Russo, "Cannabis in India."

49. Ethan B. Russo, "Taming THC: Potential Cannabis Synergy and Phytocannabinoid-Terpenoid Entourage Effects," *British Journal of Pharmacology* 163(7) (2011): 1344–1364.

50. Abigail Geiger, "Support for Marijuana Legalization Begins to Rise," Pew Research Center's Fact Tank: News in the Numbers (October 12, 2016), accessed October 31, 2017, http://www.pewresearch.org/fact-tank/2016/10/12/support-for-marijuana-legalization-continues-to-rise/.

51. John Hudak and Grace Wallack, "Ending the U.S. Government's War on Medical Marijuana Research," Report from the Brookings Institute Center for Effective Public Management, October 2015.

52. Center for Behavioral Health Statistics and Quality, "Behavioral Health Trends in the United States: Results from the 2014 National Survey on Drug Use and Health" (HHS Publication No. SMA 15–4927, NSDUH Series H-50, 2015), p. 5. For more, see http://www.drugwarfacts.org/cms/Drug_Usage#Cannabis.

53. Harold Kalant, Amy J. Porath-Waller, "Clearing the Smoke on Cannabis: Medical Use of Cannabis and Cannabinoids," Canadian Centre on Substance Abuse (CCSA), 2016. http://www.ccsa.ca/Resource%20Library/CCSA-Medical-Use-of-Cannabis-Report-2016-en.pdf, accessed November 3, 2017.

54. Mohamed Ben Amar, "Cannabinoids in Medicine: A Review of Their Therapeutic Potential," *Journal of Ethnopharmacology* 105 (1–2): 1–25, 2006.

55. Russell Noyes Jr. et al., "Analgesic Effect of Delta-9-Tetrahydrocannabinol," *Journal of Clinical Pharmacology* 15 (2–3) (February–March 1975): 139–143.

56. Drug Enforcement Administration, "The Drug Enforcement Administration Position on Marijuana, 2013," https://www.dea.gov/docs/marijuana_position_2011.pdf, accessed November 3, 2017.

57. D. J. Debono, L. J. Hoeksema, and R. D. Hobbs, "Caring for Patients with Chronic Pain: Pearls and Pitfalls," *Journal of the American Osteopathic Association* 113(8) (2013): 620–627.

58. Department of Economic and Social Affairs of the United Nations Secretariat Consolidated, "List of Products Whose Consumption and/or Sale Have Been Banned, Withdrawn, Severely Restricted or not Approved by Governments," 12th issue (New York: Pharmaceuticals United Nations, 2005).

59. Holland. "The Pot Book."

60. Thomas Bodenheimer, "Uneasy Alliance—Clinical Investigators and the Pharmaceutical Industry," *New England Journal of Medicine* 342 (May 18, 2000): 1539–1544.

61. P. C. Gotzsche, "Does Long Term Use of Psychiatric Drugs Cause More Harm Than Good?" *British Medical Journal* 350 (May 12, 2015): 2435.

62. U.S. Department of Health and Human Services, U.S. Food and Drug Administration, "Development and Approval Process (Drugs), Preventable Adverse Drug Reactions: A Focus on Drug Reactions," updated March 14, 2016.

63. Jo Marchant, *Cure: The Journey into the Science of Mind over Body,* New York: Crown Publishers, 2016.

64. Assafa Shelef et. al, "Safety and Efficacy of Medical Cannabis Oil for Behavioral and Psychological Symptoms of Dementia: An Open-Label, Add-On, Pilot Study," *Journal of Alzheimer's Disease* 51(1) (2016): 15–19.

65. Russo, Ethan B., "Cannabinoids in the Management of Difficult to Treat Pain," *Therapeutics and Clinical Risk Management* 4(1) (2008): 245–259.

66. Simone Tambaro and Marco Bortolato, "Cannabinoid-Related Agents in the Treatment of Anxiety Disorders: Current Knowledge and Future Perspectives," *Recent Patents on CNS Drug Discovery* 7(1) (2012): 25–40.

67. Luciano Rezende Vilela et al., "Cannabidiol Rescues Acute Hepatic Toxicity and Seizure Induced by Cocaine," *Mediators of Inflammation* 2015 (Article ID 523418, 12 pages, 2015).

68. R. Ader and N. Cohen, "Behaviorally Conditioned Immunosuppression," *Psychosomatic Medicine* 37(4) (July–August 1975): 333–340.

69. J. M. Williams et al., *Brain Research Bulletin* 6 (1981): 83–94.

70. A. Dietrich and W. F. McDaniel, "Endocannabinoids and Exercise," *British Journal of Sports Medicine* 38(5) (2004): 536–541.

71. E. Fride et al., "Milk Intake and Survival in Newborn Cannabinoid CB1 Receptor Knockout Mice: Evidence for a 'CB3' Receptor," *European Journal of Pharmacology* 461(1) (February 7, 2003): 27–34.

72. Johns Hopkins Medicine, "The Brain-Gut Connection: Anxiety and Depres-

sion Have Been Thought to Contribute to Gastro Conditions Like Irritable Bowel Syndrome (IBS)," johnshopkinsmedicine.org, accessed November 6, 2017.

73. Martin A Makary and Michael Daniel, "Medical Error—The Third Leading Cause of Death in the US," *British Medical Journal* 353 (May 3, 2016).

74. David Cassarett, "A Doctor's Case for Medical Marijuana," Ted.com, TEDMED, November 2016, https://www.ted.com/talks/david_casarett_a_doctor_s_case_for _medical_marijuana, accessed November 19, 2017.

75. Rupal Pandey et al., "Endocannabinoids and Immune Regulation," *Pharmacological Research: The Official Journal of the Italian Pharmacological Society* 60(2) (2009): 85–92.

76. O. Devinsky, B. J. Whalley, and V. Di Marzo, "Cannabinoids in the Treatment of Neurological Disorders," *Neurotherapeutics* 12 (2015): 689.

77. Sean D. McAllister et al., "Pathways Mediating the Effects of Cannabidiol on the Reduction of Breast Cancer Cell Proliferation, Invasion, and Metastasis," *Breast Cancer Research and Treatment* 129(1) (2011): 37–47.

78. Prakash Nagarkatti et al., "Cannabinoids as Novel Anti-Inflammatory Drugs," *Future Medicinal Chemistry* 1(7) (2009): 1333–1349.

79. Sandeep Vasant More and Dong-Kug Choi, "Promising Cannabinoid-Based Therapies for Parkinson's Disease: Motor Symptoms to Neuroprotection," *Molecular Neurodegeneration* 10 (2015): 17.

80. Torsten Lowin and Rainer H. Straub, "Cannabinoid-Based Drugs Targeting CB_1 and $TRPV_1$, the Sympathetic Nervous System, and Arthritis," *Arthritis Research & Therapy* 17(1) (2015): 226.

81. Russo, "Cannabinoids in the Management of Difficult to Treat Pain."

82. T. Naftali et al., "Cannabis Induces a Clinical Response in Patients with Crohn's Disease: A Prospective Placebo-Controlled Study," *Clinical Gastroenterol Hepatology* 11(10) (October 2013):1276–1280.

83. Centers for Disease Control and Prevention, "Understanding the Epidemic," 2016, https://www.cdc.gov/drugoverdose/epidemic/, accessed November 19, 2017.

84. Rita Paul-Sen Gupta, Margaret L. de Wit, and David McKeown, "The Impact of Poverty on the Current and Future Health Status of Children," *Paediatrics & Child Health* 12(8) (2007): 667–672.

85. Holland, *The Pot Book.*

86. Ibid.

87. D. P. Tashkin et al., "Effects of Smoked Marijuana in Experimentally Induced Asthma," *American Review of Respiratory Diseases* 112(3) (September 1975): 377–386.

88. Harvard Health Publications, Harvard Medical School, "Drugs in the Water,"

June 2011, www.health.harvard.edu/newsletter_article/drugs-in-the-water, accessed November 6, 2017.

89. "Guidelines for URA Residential and Light Commercial Zones, Northampton, Massachusetts," http://www.northampton.zone/current-zoning/, accessed November 6, 2017.

90. Dylan Matthews, "The Black/White Marijuana Arrest Gap, in Nine Charts," *Washington Post* Wonk Blog, June 4, 2013, accessed November 6, 2017.

91. Kogan and Mechoulam, "Cannabinoids in Health and Disease."

92. Drug Enforcement Administration, "Operations, Domestic Cannabis Eradication / Suppression Program," 2015, https://www.dea.gov/ops/cannabis.shtml, accessed November 6, 2017.

93. R. A. Rudd et al., "Increases in Drug and Opioid-Involved Overdose Deaths— United States 2010–2015," *Centers for Disease Control Morbidity and Mortality Weekly Report* 65 (2016): 1445–1452.

94. James B. Mowry et al., "2014 Annual Report of the American Association of Poison Control Centers' National Poison Data System (NPDS): 32nd Annual Report," *Clinical Toxicology* 53(10) (2015): 962–1146.

95. No recorded cases of overdose deaths from cannabis have been found in extensive literature reviews; see, for example, Robert S. Gable, "The Toxicity of Recreational Drugs," *American Scientist* 94(3) (May–June 2006): 207.

TWO At Their Wits' End

1. V. K. Agnihotri et al., "Therapeutic Significance of Shiroabhyanga: A Review," *International Journal of Research in Ayurveda & Pharmacy* 6(6) (November–December 2015).

2. John Douillard, *Encyclopedia of Ayurvedic Massage,* Berkeley, CA: North Atlantic Books, 2004: 14.

3. Sriranjini Sitaram Jaideep et al., "Modulation of Cardiac Autonomic Dysfunction in Ischemic Stroke following Ayurveda (Indian System of Medicine) Treatment," *Evidence-Based Complementary and Alternative Medicine* 2014 (Article ID 634695, 8 pages, 2014).

4. S. Subramaniam et al., "Bioinformatics and Systems Biology of the Lipidome," *Chemical Reviews* 111(10) (October 2011): 6452–6490.

5. A. J. Basler, "Pilot Study Investigating the Effects of Ayurvedic Abhyanga Massage on Subjective Stress Experience," *Journal of Alternative and Complementary Medicine* 17(5) (May 2011): 435–440.

6. P. Lucas, "Cannabis as an Adjunct to or Substitute for Opiates in the Treatment of Chronic Pain," *Journal of Psychoactive Drugs* 44(2) (April–June 2012): 125–133.

7. Andrew Jones, "Psychiatric Effects of Cannabis," *British Journal of Psychiatry* 178(2) (February 2001): 116–122.

8. P. Pacher, S. Bátkai, and G. Kunos, "The Endocannabinoid System as an Emerging Target of Pharmacotherapy," *Pharmacology Review* 58(3) (September 2006): 389–462.

9. Jonathan A. Galli, Ronald Andari Sawaya, and Frank K. Friedenberg, "Cannabinoid Hyperemesis Syndrome," *Current Drug Abuse Reviews* 4(4) (2011): 241–249.

10. Ethan B. Russo, "Taming THC: Potential Cannabis Synergy and Phytocannabinoid-Terpenoid Entourage Effects," *British Journal of Pharmacology* 163(7) (2011): 1344–1364.

11. Russo, "Cannabinoids in the Management of Difficult to Treat Pain."

12. J. A. Crippa et al., "Neural Basis of Anxiolytic Effects of Cannabidiol (CBD) in Generalized Social Anxiety Disorder: A Preliminary Report," *Journal of Psychopharmacology* 25(1) (January 2011):121–130.

13. S. W. Smith, M. Hauben, and J. K. Aronson, "Paradoxical and Bidirectional Drug Effects," *Drug Safety* 35(3) (March 1, 2012): 173–189.

14. Kogan and Mechoulam, "Cannabinoids in Health and Disease."

15. A. R. de Mello Schier et al., "Antidepressant-Like and Anxiolytic-Like Effects of Cannabidiol: A Chemical Compound of *Cannabis sativa*," *CNS and Neurological Disorders—Drug Targets* 13(6) (2014): 953–960.

16. Mélissa Prud'homme, Romulus Cata, and Didier Jutras-Aswad, "Cannabidiol as an Intervention for Addictive Behaviors: A Systematic Review of the Evidence," *Substance Abuse: Research and Treatment* 9 (2015): 33–38.

17. F. J. Evans, "Cannabinoids: The Separation of Central from Peripheral Effects on a Structural Basis," *Planta Medica* 57(7) (October 1991): 60–67.

18. C. E. Turner, M. A. Elsohly, and E. G. Boeren EG, "Constituents of *Cannabis sativa* L. XVII: A Review of the Natural Constituents," *Journal of Natural Products* 43(2) (March–April 1980): 169–234.

19. G. Appendino et al., "Antibacterial Cannabinoids from *Cannabis sativa*: A Structure-Activity Study," *Journal of Natural Products* 71(8) (August 2008):1427–1430.

20. R. E. Musty et al., "Interactions of Delta-9-Tetrahydrocannabinol and Cannabinol in Man," in M. C. Braude and S. Szara, eds., *The Pharmacology of Marihuana,* vol. 2 (New York: Raven Press, 1976): 559–563.

21. Russo, "Taming THC."

22. T. Komori et al., "Effects of Citrus Fragrance on Immune Function and Depressive States," *Neuroimmunomodulation* 2(3) (May–June 1995): 174–180.

23. Christelle M. Andre, Jean-Francois Hausman, and Gea Guerriero, "*Cannabis sativa:* The Plant of the Thousand and One Molecules," *Frontiers in Plant Science* 7 (2016): 19.

24. C. Blázquez et al., "Inhibition of Tumor Angiogenesis by Cannabinoids," *Federation of American Societies for Experimental Biology Journal* 17(3) (March 2003): 529–531.

25. A. Preet, R. K. Ganju, and J. E. Groopman, "Delta9-Tetrahydrocannabinol Inhibits Epithelial Growth Factor–Induced Lung Cancer Cell Migration In Vitro as Well as Its Growth and Metastasis In Vivo," *Oncogene* 27(3) (January 10, 2008): 339–346.

26. M. Guzmán et al., "A Pilot Clinical Study of Delta9-Tetrahydrocannabinol in Patients with Recurrent Glioblastoma Multiforme," *British Journal of Cancer* 95(2) (July 17, 2006): 197–203.

27. David Gorski, "Medical Marijuana as the New Herbalism, Part 2: Cannabis Does Not Cure Cancer," Science Based Medicine: Exploring Issues and Controversies in Science and Medicine, Sciencebasedmedicine.org, August 11, 2014, accessed November 10, 2017.

28. American Cancer Society, "Probability (%) of Developing Invasive Cancer during Selected Age Intervals by Sex, US, 2011–2013," Cancer Facts and Figures 2017, www.cancer.org, accessed November 10, 2017.

29. M. Guzmán, "Cannabinoids: Potential Anticancer Agents," *Nature Reviews: Cancer* 3(10) (October 2003): 745–755.

30. Tore Sanner and Tom K. Grimsrud, "Nicotine: Carcinogenicity and Effects on Response to Cancer Treatment—A Review," *Frontiers in Oncology* 5 (2015): 196.

31. World Health Organization, "Tobacco Fact Sheet," 2017, www.who.int, accessed November 10, 2017.

32. Robert Melamede, "Cannabis and Tobacco Smoke Are Not Equally Carcinogenic," *Harm Reduction Journal* 2 (2005): 21.

33. R. T. Greenlee et al., "Cancer Statistics, 2001," *CA: A Cancer Journal for Clinicians* 51 (2001): 15–36.

34. Bandana Chakravarti, Janani Ravi, and Ramesh K. Ganju, "Cannabinoids as Therapeutic Agents in Cancer: Current Status and Future Implications," *Oncotarget* 5(15) (2014): 5852–5872.

35. Rachel Sherman and John Hickner, "Academic Physicians Use Placebos in Clinical Practice and Believe in the Mind-Body Connection," *Journal of General Internal Medicine* 23(1) (2008): 7–10.

36. Sheldon Cohen and Bruce Rabin, "Psychological Stress, Immunity, and Cancer," *Journal of the National Cancer Institute* 90(1) (1998): 3–4.

37. Russo, "Cannabinoids in the Management of Difficult to Treat Pain."

38. Zoltán Járai et al., "Cannabinoid-induced Mesenteric Vasodilation through an Endothelial Site Distinct from CB1 or CB2 Receptors," *Proceedings of the National Academy of Sciences* 96(24) (1999): 14136–14141.

39. Melamede, "Cannabis and Tobacco Smoke Are Not Equally Carcinogenic."

40. Paola Massi et al., "Cannabidiol as Potential Anticancer Drug," *British Journal of Clinical Pharmacology* 75(2) (2013): 303–312.

41. G. R. Ross et al., "Evidence for the Putative Cannabinoid Receptor (GPR55)–Mediated Inhibitory Effects on Intestinal Contractility in Mice," *Pharmacology* 90(1–2) (2012): 55–65.

42. Barry Marshall and Paul C Adams, "*Helicobacter pylori:* A Nobel Pursuit?" *Canadian Journal of Gastroenterology* 22(11) (2008): 895–896.

43. Loraine D. Marrett et al., "Cancer in Canada in 2008," *CMAJ: Canadian Medical Association Journal* 179(11) (2008): 1163–1170.

THREE What about the Children?

1. C. Jones, "Sources of Prescription Opioid Pain Relievers by Frequency of Past Year Nonmedical Use: United States, 2008 to 2011," *Journal of the American Medical Association: International Medicine* 174(5) (2014): 802–803.

2. R. A. Rudd et al., "Increases in Drug and Opioid-Involved Overdose Deaths—United States, 2010–2015," *Centers for Disease Control Morbidity and Mortality Weekly Report* 65(50–51) (December 30, 2016): 1445–1452.

3. U.S. Department of Health and Human Services, Substance Abuse and Mental Health Services Administration, "Highlights of the 2011 Drug Abuse Warning Network (DAWN) Findings on Drug-Related Emergency Department Visits," the DAWN Report, February 22, 2013.

4. J. A. Boscarino et al., "Risk Factors for Drug Dependence among Out-Patients on Opioid Therapy in a Large US Health-Care System," *Addiction* 105 (October 2010): 1776–1782.

5. P. Robson, "Abuse Potential and Psychoactive Effects of δ-9-Tetrahydrocannabinol and Cannabidiol Oromucosal Spray (Sativex), a New Cannabinoid Medicine," *Expert Opinion on Drug Safety* 10(5) (September 2011): 675–685.

6. F. A. Wagner and J. C. Anthony, "From First Drug Use to Drug Dependence: Developmental Periods of Risk for Dependence upon Marijuana, Cocaine, and Alcohol," *Neuropsychopharmacology* 26(4) (April 2002): 479–488.

7. Martin A. Makary and Michael Daniel, "Medical Error: The Third Leading Cause of Death in the US," *British Medical Journal* 353 (2016).

8. George Sam Wang et al., "Unintentional Pediatric Exposures to Marijuana in Colorado, 2009–2015," *Journal of the American Medical Association: Pediatrics* 170(9) (2016): e160971.

9. I. Galve-Roperh et al., "Cannabinoid Receptor Signaling in Progenitor/Stem Cell Proliferation and Differentiation," *Progress in Lipid Research* 52(4) (October 2013): 633–650.

10. E. Fride, "Multiple Roles for the Endocannabinoid System during the Earliest Stages of Life: Pre- and Postnatal Development," *Journal of Neuroendocrinology* 20 (May 2008, Supplement 1): 75–81.

11. Ibid.

12. E. Fride, "The Endocannabinoid-CB Receptor System: Importance for Development and in Pediatric Disease," *Neuro Endocrinology Letters* 25(1–2) (February–April 2004): 24–30.

13. National Institute on Drug Abuse (NIDA), "Fentanyl," June 3, 2016, https://www.drugabuse.gov/publications/drugfacts/fentanyl, accessed November 11, 2017.

14. World Health Organization, "WHO Model List of Essential Medicines (20th List)," March 2017, http://www.who.int/medicines/publications/essentialmedicines /en/, accessed November 10, 2017.

15. United Nations Office on Drugs and Crime, Commission on Narcotic Drugs Press Release, "Commission on Narcotic Drugs Takes Decisive Step to Help Prevent Deadly Fentanyl Overdoses," March 16, 2017, www.unodc.org, accessed November 10, 2017.

16. Nahid Jahani Shoorab et al., "The Effect of Intravenous Fentanyl on Pain and Duration of the Active Phase of First Stage Labor," *Oman Medical Journal* 28(5) (2013): 306–310.

17. Claire Shannon et al., "Placental Transfer of Fentanyl in Early Human Pregnancy," *Human Reproduction* 13(8) (1998): 2317–2320.

18. American Pregnancy Association, "Using Narcotics for Pain Relief during Childbirth: Types and Side Effects," http://americanpregnancy.org/labor-and-birth /narcotics/, accessed November 10, 2017.

19. Christopher McPherson and Ruth E. Grunau, "Neonatal Pain Control and Neurologic Effects of Anesthetics and Sedatives in Preterm Infants," *Clinics in Perinatology* 41(1) (2014): 209–227.

20. Steven Nelson, "Fentanyl Maker Donates Big to Campaign Opposing Pot Legalization," *U.S. News and World Report,* September 8, 2016, https://www.usnews .com, accessed November 10, 2017.

21. Lucas, "Cannabis as an Adjunct to or Substitute for Opiates."

22. Tambaro and Bortolato, "Cannabinoid-Related Agents."

23. L. Hanuš et al., "HU-308: A Specific Agonist for CB_2, a Peripheral Cannabinoid Receptor," *Proceedings of the National Academy of Sciences of the United States of America* 96(25) (1999): 14228–14233.

24. Michael Camilleri, "Opioid-Induced Constipation: Challenges and Therapeutic Opportunities," *American Journal of Gastroenterology* 106 (2011): 835–842.

25. Alfred D. Nelson and Michael Camilleri, "Chronic Opioid Induced Constipation in Patients with Nonmalignant Pain: Challenges and Opportunities," *Therapeutic Advances in Gastroenterology* 8(4) (2015): 206–220.

26. Fride, "The Endocannabinoid-CB Receptor System."

27. Jayleen K. L. Gunn et al., "The Effects of Prenatal Cannabis Exposure on Fetal Development and Pregnancy Outcomes: A Protocol," *British Medical Journal* 5(3) (2015): e007227, http://bmjopen.bmj.com/content/5/3/e007227, accessed November 20, 2017.

28. E. E Hatch and M. B. Bracken, "Effect of Cannabis Use in Pregnancy on Fetal Growth," *American Journal of Epidemiology* 124 (1986): 986–993.

29. Gunn et al., "The Effects of Prenatal Cannabis Exposure on Fetal Development."

30. Hatch and Bracken, "Effect of Cannabis Use in Pregnancy on Fetal Growth."

31. M. C. Dreher, K. Nugent, and R. Hudgins, "Prenatal Marijuana Exposure and Neonatal Outcomes in Jamaica: An Ethnographic Study," *Pediatrics* 93(2) (February 1994): 254–260.

32. Ibid.

33. National Academies of Sciences, Engineering, and Medicine, "Prenatal, Perinatal, and Neonatal Exposure to Cannabis," in *The Health Effects of Cannabis and Cannabinoids: The Current State of Evidence and Recommendations for Research* (Washington, DC: National Academies Press, 2017), https://www.ncbi.nlm.nih.gov/books/NBK425751/, accessed November 20, 2017.

34. Medicine.net, Pregnancy, "Dangerous Drugs for Baby," https://www.medicine net.com/script/main/art.asp?articlekey=9337, accessed November 10, 2017.

35. Cable News Network (CNN), "Marijuana Stops Child's Severe Seizures," August 7, 2013, http://www.cnn.com/2013/08/07/health/charlotte-child-medical-marijuana/, accessed November 10, 2017.

36. This is not a scientific statement but comes from an Ayurvedic medicinal principle that nutrients take about thirty days to be absorbed into and penetrate all tissue layers.

37. Ralph Hingson and Donald Kenkel, "Social, Health, and Economic Consequences of Underage Drinking," in Richard J. Bonnie and Mary Ellen O'Connell, eds.,

Reducing Underage Drinking: A Collective Responsibility (Washington, DC: National Academies Press, 2003), https://www.ncbi.nlm.nih.gov/books/NBK37611/, accessed November 20, 2017.

38. A. D. Manthripragada et al., "Characterization of Acetaminophen Overdose–Related Emergency Department Visits and Hospitalizations in the United States," *Pharmacoepidemiology and Drug Safety* 20(8) (August 2011): 819–826.

39. National Institute on Drug Abuse, "Cough and Cold Medicine Abuse," May 2014, https://www.drugabuse.gov/publications/drugfacts/cough-cold-medicine -abuse, accessed November 10, 2017.

40. National Institute on Alcohol Abuse and Alcoholism, "Alcohol Facts and Statistics," https://www.niaaa.nih.gov/alcohol-health/overview-alcohol-consumption /alcohol-facts-and-statistics, accessed November 20, 2017.

41. Rainer J. Klement and Ulrike Kämmerer, "Is There a Role for Carbohydrate Restriction in the Treatment and Prevention of Cancer?" *Nutrition & Metabolism* 8 (2011): 75.

42. Katherine Esposito and Dario Giugliano, "Diet and Inflammation: A Link to Metabolic and Cardiovascular Diseases," *European Heart Journal* 27(1) (2006): 15–20.

43. John Ingold, "Kids' Emergency Room Visits for Marijuana Increased in Colorado after Legalization, Study Finds; Edibles Account for Nearly Half of Accidental Exposures,"

Denver Post, October 2, 2016, www.denverpost.com, accessed November 10, 2017.

44. Harumi Ikei, Chorong Song, and Yoshifumi Miyazaki, "Effects of Olfactory Stimulation by α-pinene on Autonomic Nervous Activity," *Journal of Wood Science* 62(6) (December 2016): 568–572.

45. Food Safety News, "Third Death in Colorado Linked to Marijuana Edibles," March 27, 2015, www.foodsafetynews.com/2015/03/third-death-in-colorado -linked-to-edible-marijuana/#.WIfEZpK1LW, accessed November 12, 2017.

46. Ibid.

FOUR Young Adults

Epigraph: William Mackworth Young, *Report of the Indian Hemp Drugs Commission 1893–94,* vol. 1 (London: Hardinge Simpole Publishing, 2010).

. Kathrin F. Stanger-Hall and David W. Hall, "Abstinence-Only Education and Teen Pregnancy Rates: Why We Need Comprehensive Sex Education in the U.S.," *Public Library of Science (PLOS) One* 6(10) (2011): e24658.

2. Richard A. Grucza et al., "Declining Prevalence of Marijuana Use Disorders

among Adolescents in the United States, 2002 to 2013," *Child and Adolescent Psychiatry* 55(6) (June 2016): 487–494.

3. Deborah S. Hasin, "Medical Marijuana Laws and Adolescent Marijuana Use in the USA from 1991 to 2014: Results from Annual, Repeated Cross-Sectional Surveys," *Lancet Psychiatry* 2 (2015): 601–608.

4. L. D. Johnston et al., *Monitoring the Future: National Survey Results on Drug Use, 1975–2014—2014 Overview: Key Findings on Adolescent Drug Use,* Ann Arbor: Institute for Social Research, University of Michigan, 2015.

5. Michael McKinney, "Rhode Island State Rep. Edith Ajello Says Studies Indicate Minors Find It Easier to Get Marijuana Than Alcohol," Politifact.com, February 16, 2013, accessed November 12, 2017.

6. Monte Whaley, "Colorado Districts Wrestle with New Law Allowing Students to Use Medical Marijuana at School," *Denver Post,* August 22, 2016.

7. The Cannabist, "Disabled Teen Can't Have Cannabis Treatments While at Jeffco School," *Denver Post,* February 10, 2015.

8. Irving Kirsch, "Antidepressants and the Placebo Effect," *Zeitschrift für Psychologie* 222(3) (2014): 128–134.

9. Jack Alan McCain, "Antidepressants and Suicide in Adolescents and Adults: A Public Health Experiment with Unintended Consequences?" *Pharmacy and Therapeutics* 34(7) (2009): 355–378.

10. Yasmina Molero et al., "Selective Serotonin Reuptake Inhibitors and Violent Crime: A Cohort Study," *Public Library of Science Medicine* 12(9) (September 15, 2015), https://www.ncbi.nlm.nih.gov/pubmed/26372359, accessed November 20, 2017.

11. Peter R. Breggin, "Suicidality, Violence and Mania Caused by Selective Serotonin Reuptake Inhibitors (SSRIs): A Review and Analysis," *International Journal of Risk & Safety in Medicine* 16 (2003/2004): 31–49.

12. Yasmina Molero et al., "Selective Serotonin Reuptake Inhibitors and Violent Crime."

13. Jeffrey Susman and Brian Klee, "The Role of High-Potency Benzodiazepines in the Treatment of Panic Disorder," *Primary Care Companion to the Journal of Clinical Psychiatry* 7(1) (2005): 5–11.

14. J. O. Cole and J. C. Kando, "Adverse Behavioral Events Reported in Patients Taking Alprazolam and Other Benzodiazepines," *Journal of Clinical Psychiatry* 54(10 Supplement) (1993): 49–63.

15. Lex Wunderink et al., "Recovery in Remitted First-Episode Psychosis at 7

Years of Follow-up of an Early Dose Reduction/Discontinuation or Maintenance Treatment Strategy; Long-Term Follow-up of a 2-Year Randomized Clinical Trial," *Journal of the American Medical Association Psychiatry* 70(9) (September 2013): 913–920.

16. J. Moncrieff, "Does Antipsychotic Withdrawal Provoke Psychosis? Review of the Literature on Rapid Onset Psychosis (Supersensitivity Psychosis) and Withdrawal-Related Relapse," *Acta Psychiatrica Scandinavica* 114(1) (July 2006): 3–13.

17. Alejandro Aparisi Rey et al., "Biphasic Effects of Cannabinoids in Anxiety Responses: CB1 and GABA$_B$ Receptors in the Balance of GABAergic and Glutamatergic Neurotransmission," *Neuropsychopharmacology* 37(12) (2012): 2624–2634.

18. Lex Pelger, "The Endocannabinoid System: Deep Dive," Holistic Cannabis Academy Lecture, Track III, Module 1, 2016.

19. Madeline H. Meier, "Persistent Cannabis Users Show Neuropsychological Decline from Childhood to Midlife," *Proceedings of the National Academy of Sciences* 109(40): E2657–E2664.

20. Nicholas J. Jackson, "Impact of Adolescent Marijuana Use on Intelligence: Results from Two Longitudinal Twin Studies," *Proceedings of the National Academy of Sciences* 113(5): E500–E508.

21. Jodi M. Gilman et. al., "Cannabis Use Is Quantitatively Associated with Nucleus Accumbens and Amygdala Abnormalities in Young Adult Recreational Users," *Journal of Neuroscience* 34(16) (April 16, 2014): 5529–5538.

22. J. Weiland et al., "Daily Marijuana Use Is Not Associated with Brain Morphometric Measures in Adolescents or Adults," *Journal of Neuroscience* 35(4) (January 28, 2015): 1505–1512.

23. S. A. Gruber et. al., "Splendor in the Grass? A Pilot Study Assessing the Impact of Medical Marijuana on Executive Function," *Frontiers in Pharmacology* 7(355) (October 13, 2016), https://www.ncbi.nlm.nih.gov/pubmed/27790138, accessed November 20, 2017.

24. Zerrin Atakan, "Cannabis, a Complex Plant: Different Compounds and Different Effects on Individuals," *Therapeutic Advances in Psychopharmacology* 2(6) (2012): 241–254.

25. Personal e-mail correspondence with Ken Snoke, "Post MJbizconference questions," June 14, 2015.

26. Javier Iribarren et al., "Post-Traumatic Stress Disorder: Evidence-Based Research for the Third Millennium," *Evidence-Based Complementary and Alternative Medicine* 2(4) (2005): 503–512.

27. Tabea Schoeler and Sagnik Bhattacharyya, "The Effect of Cannabis Use on Memory Function: An Update," *Substance Abuse and Rehabilitation* 4 (2013): 11–27.

28. B. M. Nguyen et al., "Effect of Marijuana Use on Outcomes in Traumatic Brain Injury, *American Surgeon* 80(10) (October 2014): 979–983.

29. Ayelet Cohen-Yeshurun et al., "*N*-Arachidonoyl-L-Serine (AraS) Possesses Proneurogenic Properties *in Vitro* and *in Vivo* after Traumatic Brain Injury," *Journal of Cerebral Blood Flow & Metabolism* 33(8) (2013): 1242–1250.

30. Wen Jiang et al., "Cannabinoids Promote Embryonic and Adult Hippocampus Neurogenesis."

31. Bryan Kolb, Robbin Gibb, and Terry Robinson, "Brain Plasticity and Behavior," Canadian Centre for Behavioural Neuroscience, University of Lethbridge, Alberta, Canada, and Department of Psychology, University of Michigan, Ann Arbor, https://www.psychologicalscience.org/journals/cd/12_1/Kolb.cfm, accessed November 20, 2017.

32. Meng Li, Jun Liu, and Joe Z. Tsien, "Theory of Connectivity: Nature and Nurture of Cell Assemblies and Cognitive Computation," *Frontiers in Neural Circuits* 10 (2016): 34.

33. Wilson M. Compton, "Marijuana Use and Use Disorders in Adults in the USA, 2002–14: Analysis of Annual Cross-Sectional Surveys," *Lancet Psychiatry* 3(10) (August 31, 2016): 954–964.

34. National Institute on Alcohol Abuse and Alcoholism, "Alcohol Use Disorder," 2012, www.niaaa.nih.gov/alcohol-health/overview-alcohol-consumption/alcohol-use-disorders, accessed November 12, 2017.

35. Rajiv Radhakrishnan, Samuel T. Wilkinson, and Deepak Cyril D'Souza, "Gone to Pot—A Review of the Association between Cannabis and Psychosis," *Frontiers in Psychiatry* 5 (2014): 54.

36. H. Hafner, "Are Mental Disorders Increasing over Time?" *Psychopathology* 18(2–3) (1985): 66–81.

37. J. Rentzsch et al., "Differential Impact of Heavy Cannabis Use on Sensory Gating in Schizophrenic Patients and Otherwise Healthy Controls," *Experimental Neurology* 205(1) (2007): 241–249.

38. E. Moore, "The Impact of Alcohol and Illicit Drugs on People with Psychosis," *Australia New Zealand Journal of Psychiatry* 46(9) (September 2012): 864–878.

39. J. Rentzsch et al., "Differential Impact of Heavy Cannabis Use."

40. Carissa M. Coulstona et al., "The Neuropsychological Correlates of Cannabis Use in Schizophrenia: Lifetime Abuse/Dependence, Frequency of Use, and Recency of Use," *Schizophrenia Research* 96(1–3) (November 2007): 169–184.

41. Agrawal Divya et al., "Split Brain Syndrome: One Brain but Two Conscious Minds?" *Journal of Health Research and Reviews* 1(2) (2014): 27–33.

42. Yasmina Molero et al., "Selective Serotonin Reuptake Inhibitors and Violent Crime."

43. Kathryn A. Roecklein and Kelly J. Rohan, "Seasonal Affective Disorder: An Overview and Update," *Psychiatry (Edgmont)* 2(1) (2005): 20–26.

44. L. Edwards and P. Torcellini, *A Literature Review of the Effects of Natural Light on Building Occupants,* Golden, CO: Natural Renewable Energy Laboratory, July 2002, https://www.nrel.gov/docs/fy02osti/30769.pdf, accessed November 20, 2017.

FIVE The Cannabis Householder

1. Drug Enforcement Administration, "Domestic Cannabis Eradication / Suppression Program," 2016, https://www.dea.gov/ops/cannabis.shtml, accessed November 20, 2017.

2. L. W. Buckalew and S. Ross, "Relationship of Perceptual Characteristics to Efficacy of Placebos," *Psychological Reports* 49(3) (December 1981): 955–961.

3. Denis Romero, "Marijuana Strains Like OG Kush Are Meaningless, Expert Says," *LA Weekly,* Tuesday, December 3, 2013, www.laweekly.com, accessed November 12, 2017.

4. Stevan Harnad, "How/Why the Mind-Body Problem Is Hard," *Journal of Consciousness Studies* 7(4) (April 2000): 54–61.

5. I. Matias et. al., "Occurrence and Possible Biological Role of the Endocannabinoid System in the Sea Squirt *Ciona intestinali*," *Journal of Neurochemistry* 93(5) (June 2005): 1141–1156.

6. J. M. McPartland and G. W. Guy, "The Evolution of Cannabis and Coevolution with the Cannabinoid Receptor—A Hypothesis," in G. W. Guy, B. A. Whittle, and P. J. Robson, eds., *The Medicinal Uses of Cannabinoids,* 71–101 (London, Chicago: Pharmaceutical Press).

7. Marchant, *Cure.*

8. E. Ali et al., "Antimicrobial Activity of *Cannabis sativa* L.," *Chinese Medicine* 3(1) (2012): 61–64.

9. John Lydo et. al., "Uv-B Radiation Effects on Photosynthesis, Growth and Cannabinoid Production of Two *Cannabis sativa* Chemotypes," *Photochemistry and Photobiology* 46(2) (1987): 201–206.

10. D. J. Potter, "The Propagation, Characterisation and Optimisation of *Cannabis sativa* L. as a Phytopharmaceutical," PhD dissertation, King's College, London, 2009.

11. Alexander Alexandrovich Antonov, "Hidden Multiverse: Explanation of Dark Matter and Dark Energy Phenomena," *International Journal of Physics* 3(2) (2015): 84–87. http://pubs.sciepub.com/ijp/3/2/6.

12. Sam Harris et al., "The Neural Correlates of Religious and Nonreligious Belief," *Public Library of Science One* 5(1) (January 14, 2010): 10.1371, http://journals.plos.org /plosone/article?id=10.1371/annotation/7f0b174d-ab93–4844–8305–1de22836aab8, accessed November 20, 2017.

13. "Guidelines for URA Residential and Light Commercial Zones, Northampton."

14. U.S. Department of Health and Human Services, Agency for Healthcare Research and Quality, "The Number of Practicing Primary Care Physicians in the United States, 2010," https://www.ahrq.gov/research/findings/factsheets/primary/pcwork1 /index.html, accessed November 12, 2017.

15. Marijuana Business Daily, *Marijuana Business Factbook 2017: Exclusive Financial Data for Cannabusinesses & Major Investors,* MJBizFactbook.com, accessed November 20, 2017.

16. "UC Davis Study Finds Mold, Bacterial Contaminants in Medical Marijuana Samples: Immunocompromised Patients Warned about Dangers of Smoking, Vaping," UC Davis Comprehensive Cancer Center News, February 7, 2017.

17. Personal e-mail exchange with D. Andrews, November 12, 2017.

18. Marijuana Business Daily, *Marijuana Business Factbook 2017.*

19. Government of Canada, "Legalizing and Strictly Regulating Cannabis: The Facts," https://www.canada.ca/en/services/health/campaigns/legalizing-strictly -regulating-cannabis-facts.html, accessed November 12, 2017.

20. Ibid.

21. Gwen Ackerman, "Want to Research Medical Marijuana? Israel Is Open for Business: Medical Marijuana Research Takes off in Israel," Bloomberg.com/news, December 12, 2016, accessed November 12, 2017.

22. Debra Borchardt, "Marijuana Sales Totaled $6.7 Billion In 2016," *Forbes Magazine,* January 3, 2017, www.forbes.com, accessed November 12, 2017.

23. Jeffrey Miron and Katherine Waldock, "The Budgetary Impact of Ending Drug Prohibition," Cato Institute, September 27, 2010.

24. Curtis S. Florence et al., "The Economic Burden of Prescription Opioid Overdose, Abuse, and Dependence in the United States, 2013," *Medical Care* 54 (10) (2016): 901.

25. National Bureau of Economic Research, "Do Medical Marijuana Laws Reduce Addictions and Deaths Related to Pain Killers?" NBER Working Paper No. 21345, 2015.

26. CBS News, "Majority of Americans Now Support Legal Pot, Poll Says," January 23, 2014, www.cbsnews.com, accessed November 12, 2017.

27. Harborside, Oakland, CA, https://www.shopharborside.com/about/mission.html, accessed November 12, 2017.

28. Deborah S Hasin et al., "Medical Marijuana Laws and Adolescent Marijuana Use in the USA from 1991 to 2014: Results from Annual, Repeated Cross-Sectional Surveys," *Lancet Psychiatry* June 15, 2015, http://www.thelancet.com/journals/lanpsy/article/PIIS2215-0366(15)00217-5/abstract, accessed November 20, 2017.

29. Julian Santaella-Tenorio et al., "US Traffic Fatalities, 1985–2014, and Their Relationship to Medical Marijuana Laws," *American Journal of Public Health* 107(2) (February 2017): 336–342.

30. Brian Heuberger, "Despite Claims, Data Show Legalized Marijuana Has Not Increased Crime Rates," *Colorado Politics,* March 22, 2017, https://coloradopolitics.com/despite-claims-data-show-legalized-marijuana-not-increased-crime-rates/, accessed November 12, 2017.

31. Procon.org, "35 FDA-Approved Prescription Drugs Later Pulled from the Market,"

http://prescriptiondrugs.procon.org/view.resource.php?resourceID=005528, accessed November 12, 2017.

32. Rita Rubin, "How Did Vioxx Debacle Happen?" *USA Today,* October 12, 2004, A1.

33. Dr. Dustin Sulak, "Clinical Benefits of CBD," paper delivered at 4th Annual World Cannabis and Business Conference, Boston, 2017.

34. Ian Urbina, "Think Those Chemicals Have Been Tested?" *New York Times,* April 13, 2013.

35. Unitarian Universalist Association, "Alternatives to the War on Drugs, Statement of Conscience, 2002," http://www.uua.org/action/statements/alternatives-war-drugs, accessed November 12, 2017.

36. National Organization for the Reform of Marijuana Laws, "Principles of Responsible Use," www.norml.org, accessed November 12, 2017.

37. Kristen Gwynne, "Ten Worst Sentences for Marijuana-Related Crimes," Salon.com, October 29, 2012, accessed November 12, 2017.

38. Matthew G. Kirkpatrick et al., "Comparison of Intranasal Methamphetamine and *d*-Amphetamine Self-Administration by Humans," *Addiction* (Abingdon, England) 107(4) (2012): 783–791.

39. Jeremy White et al., "The Top 1 Percent: What Jobs Do They Have?" *New York Times Business,* January 15, 2012.

Index

Anslinger, Harry, 16

antinausea effects, 16, 25, 68

anxiety: antianxiety effects, 10, 28, 80, 131, 135–36; anxiety-inducing effects, 35, 67–68; physiology of, 69

aphrodisiac effects, 14

Arkansas, 175

asthma, 38, 78, 80

attention deficit/hyperactivity disorder (ADD/ADHD), 10

autism, 113–19

Ayurvedic traditional model, 9–11, 13, 58–60, 155–56, 183

Bennett, Chris, 12

Bob (consulting client), 40–41

body care products (safety of), 179

brain: Alzheimer's disease, 28; aromas and, 72; cannabis alleged effect on, 4, 16, 28, 68, 89–90, 108–10; cannabis memory effects, 38; CBD psycho-activity and, 70–71; children's brain development, 88–90, 109–10, 178; chronic traumatic encephalopathy (CTE), 124; immune system and, 29–30, 55; neurotransmitter effects on, 27–28; pain relief and, 66; schizophrenia, 136–38; teen brain debate, 119–20, 125–30; thinking/representation and, 164–67; trau-matic brain injury, 86, 88, 123–25. *See also* psychotropic and physiological effects

Bruce (consulting garden manager), 46–47

bud tenders: background and function of, 18; as community information

resource, 22; lack of medical knowledge, 7, 67, 181, 183; oversight of medicinal sales, 182; personal empowerment in healing and, 29–31

caffeine, 88

California: absence of dosing guidelines, 121–22; home grower restrictions, 18–19; legal possession regulation, 175; medical marijuana research program, 19; Proposition 215, 16–18; provision for sharing, 57; reduction in opioid prescriptions, 65; rules for caregivers, 18

Canada, 177

cancer treatment: chemotherapy origins, 78–79; dosing for, 60–63; early medicinal cannabis use for, 16; patients as cannabis advocates, 41–42; patient views of cannabis, 81–82; reduction of tumors, 20, 35, 74–78, 142; relief from symptoms and treatment effects, 25, 141; research evidence on, 73–81; sugar and, 101–2

cannabinoids. *See* CBC; CBD; CBG; CBN; limonene; terpenes; THC; THCV

cannabis history, 9–11

cannabis householders: approach to cultivation, 142–51; approach to medicinal properties, 151–54; Ayurvedic traditional model and, 155–56; as cannabis advocates, 183–84; dispensaries' relationship with, 182–83; fear of discovery, 156–63; holistic approach and,

141–42, 163–64; overview, 6. *See also* consultants

Cannabis indica. See indica

Cannabis ruderalis, 13

Cannabis sativa. See sativa

caretakers, 64

Cassarett, David, 2–3, 30

Cathy (consulting client), 133

CBC, 72

CBD (cannabidiol): antianxiety effects, 135–36; Ayurvedic references to, 10; and overdose experience, 70–71; CBD-THC entourage effect, 21, 68, 92–94; cultivation and, 69–70, 181; helicopter raid of 2015 and, 48, 174; legalization of, 7; suppression of addiction cravings, 71

CBG, 72

CBN (cannabinol), 71–72

Centers for Disease Control, 84

Cheech and Chong, 24

children: as cancer patients, 77–78; cannabis dangers to, 51; cannabis edibles and, 85, 101–2; cannabis education and, 6–7, 23, 100–101; in cannabis households, 49–51, 94–98, 171–72; cannabis packaging and, 17, 100–101; childbirth pain treatment, 86–91; childhood trauma, 125–30; conventional drugs and, 51, 83, 98; developmental plateau model and, 127–30; dispensaries and, 100–101; effect of criminalization on, 23, 40, 48–52; endocannabinoids in pregnancy and nursing, 20, 85, 88; low birth weight, 87–89; medicinal cannabis use by, 22, 24; preteen

clients, 94–101; school-based drug education, 27; teen brain debate, 119–20, 125–30; teen clients, 107–19; teen recreational users, 108–9, 125–30, 179; toddlers as clients, 91–94

China, 9

chiropractors, 183

chronic traumatic encephalopathy (CTE), 124

cocaine, 19

Colorado, 10–11, 18, 85, 102, 105–6, 109, 175, 177

Connecticut, 18, 19

consultants (cannabis consultants): account of launch experience, 32–33, 36–37; "big marijuana" influence and, 181; caretaker needs and, 64; culture of intimacy, 142–43; dispensaries' relationship with, 182–83; local business ordinances and, 39–40; police officers as clients, 43; practicing in the open, 42, 45–49, 57; referrals from medical practitioners, 57. *See also* cannabis householders; growers

convulsions, 71–72

Corey (consulting client), 117–19

criminalization (of cannabis): banks and financial services and, 175; cannabis advocacy and, 37–39; cannabis strain names and, 145–46; as deterrent to research, 24–25; "drugs" term and, 30; effect on teen users, 109; fear of discovery, 157–63; grower-police relationship, 167–68, 186; home grower restrictions, 18–19; international accounts of, 9–10;

maximum THC regulations, 17–18; overdose experiences, 70–71, 102–6; smoking as delivery method, 65–66, 115; topical oil, 59, 63, 66, 71. *See also* smoking

Dowd, Maureen, 10–12, 12

Dreher, Melanie, 89

drug dealers: as community resources, 23; dispensaries as alternative, 6; home growers as, 5; shady reputation of, 1. *See also* dispensaries

edibles: cancer treatment and, 41; commercial cannabis candy, 85; historic hash candies, 14; sugary treats as cannabis medium, 101–2, 105–6

education: bud tender training, 22; cannabis schools and training, 181; dispensaries as community information centers, 18; holistic cannabis paradigm and, 1–2, 22–23, 167; medical marijuana research program, 19; medical training, 20

Ending the U.S. Government's War on Medical Marijuana Research (Brookings Institute), 24–25

endocannabinoid system (ECS): CB1/CB2 receptors, 29, 80; evolution of, 165; fetal development of, 85; immune system connections, 29; medical training on, 24; research on, 19–20, 77, 178–79; stress reduction and, 38, 69

entourage effect, 21, 68, 92–94

epilepsy, 12, 91

Eric (consulting client), 113–17

FDA (Food and Drug Administration): anticancer drugs, 76; antipsychotic drugs, 117; approved pain medications, 4–5; cannabis testing difficulties and, 21, 81; consciousness-shifting drugs and, 167; harmful drugs approved by, 26–27, 47, 51, 84–85, 90–91, 179; holistic healing and, 167; medical advice and, 40, 168; public trust and, 30, 189; rescheduling and, 25

fentanyl, 86–87, 90

Finn, Bill, 45

Florida, 175–76

"gateway drug" designation, 16

giggling, 10, 64

growers (home growers): agency in healing and, 139–40; cannabis cultivation, 142–51; cannabis varieties and, 156–57; cloning and genetic banking, 143–44; description of cannabis garden, 33–34, 44; dispensaries' effect on, 6; as drug dealers, 5; energy consumption, 160–61; fear of discovery, 157–63; home grower experiences, 146–51, 156–57; home grower restrictions, 18; home growing legalization, 23, 139; hydroponic cultivation, 31, 148; in low-income neighborhoods, 190; outdoor growing, 44–46, 148–49, 161–63; overabundance experiences, 163–64; raids of home growers, 4, 6, 19, 26, 48; relationship with police, 167–68, 186; restrictions and criminalization, 18–19. *See also* cannabis householders; consultants; helicopter raid of 2015

cooking effect on, 118–19; drug
testing and, 186–87; in hashish,
66; Oregon maximum THC
regulations, 17–18; THCA glycerin
tincture, 115
THCV, 72
tobacco, 19
traumatic brain injury (TBI), 123–25
trichomes, 154, 166

United States Pharmacopeia, 26
University of Mississippi, 15, 24

Uruguay, 176–77
U.S. Department of Agriculture, 15, 24

war on drugs. *See* criminalization
Washington, George, 13
wasting syndrome, 25, 85
Wendy (consulting client), 170
Will (consulting client), 151–54
World Health Organization, 86

Young, Lee (consulting client), 73,
78–81